making natural

liquid
soaps

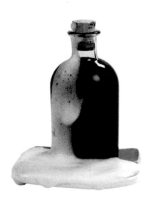

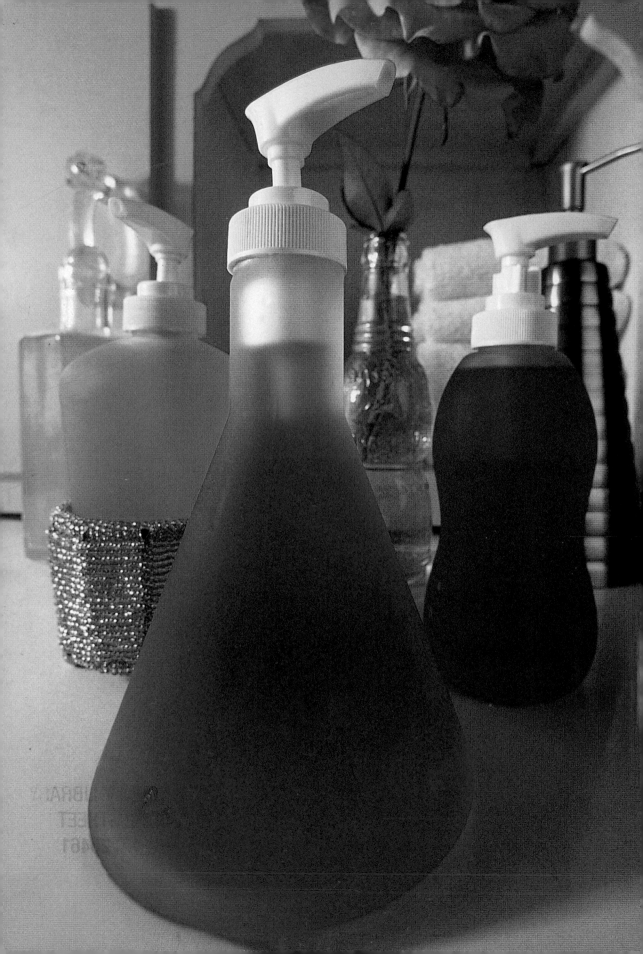

making natural
liquid soaps

herbal shower gels • conditioning shampoos
moisturizing hand soaps • luxurious bubble baths,
and more...

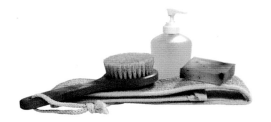

catherine failor

STOREY BOOKS

North Adams
Massachusetts

Dedicated to K. D. Grace

Many thanks to the people who have given me emotional support, offered a helping hand, and/or shed a little light: Kay Whaley, Clyde Abston, Carla Dunn, Jim Morgan, Luis Spitz, David Woodward, "Dr. Bob" McDaniel, Ray Linke, Alan Zell, and the late Jim Bronner.

The mission of Storey Publishing is to serve our customers by publishing practical information that encourages personal independence in harmony with the environment.

Edited by Deborah Balmuth and Robin Catalano
Cover design by Carol Jessop, Black Trout Design
Cover and interior photographs by Giles Prett except those by
© Jeff Burke and Lorraine Triolo for Artville on pages 91, 93, 94, 95, and 98;
© Eyewire Images on pages vii, 32, 38, 39, 40, 53, 66, 67, 92, and 134;
© PhotoDisc, Inc. on pages 48, 55, 59, 65, 76, 84, 87, 92, and 115
Text design and production by Mark Tomasi
Production assistance by Susan Bernier
Indexed by Barbara Hagerty

Copyright © 2000 by Catherine Failor

Printed in Hong Kong by C & C Offset Printing Co., Ltd
10 9 8 7 6 5 4

Library of Congress Cataloging-in-Publication Data
Failor, Catherine
    Making natural liquid soaps / Catherine Failor.
       p.   cm.
    ISBN 1-58017-243-1 (pbk. : alk. paper)
    1. Soap.   I. Title
TP991.F26   2000
668'.12—dc21
                                          99-057462
                                                  CIP

Preface

My love affair with soapmaking began more than twenty years ago when I stepped into a small bookstore in Eugene, Oregon. A slender, charming little book immediately caught my eye; the cover photo showed a woman carving designs into bars of soap. The book was *Soap: Making It, Enjoying It*, by Ann Bramson. As I stared at those bars on the cover, they seemed to me more beautiful than precious jewels. I've been making soap ever since.

I've often wondered just what it is about soapmaking that's held my attention for all these years. In part, it's because soap is so aesthetically pleasing. I never seem to tire of making it and marveling at it. But perhaps an even bigger attraction for me is that soapmaking offers so many avenues of inquiry, discovery, and invention — a seemingly endless amount!

Considering how ubiquitous soap is and what an intimate role it plays in our everyday lives, relatively little has been written about it. Compare that to cooking; gardening; or other crafts, such as sewing, jewelry making, or ceramics. Perhaps this is because soapmakers historically fell into two classes: rural women who produced "true grit" lye soap (which removed not only dirt and grime but the epidermis as well) and commercial soapmakers, whose soapmaking techniques became trade secrets.

Several excellent soapmaking books published over the past few years have helped turn the tide and refine the art of home soapmaking. All these books have been about cold-process soapmaking. But I always have an eye out for what's *not* there, which is partly a personal bent and partly a businessperson's survival reflex. And what's *not* there is information about hot-process soapmaking and all the soaps that can be made with that technique: transparent and translucent bars, liquids and gels, cream and floating soap, and more.

I first explored hot processing in my book *Making Transparent Soap* (Storey Books, 2000). *Making Natural Liquid Soaps* is a cumulation of almost two years of perspiration and further experimentation with hot-process soapmaking. Emphasis is on the perspiration — because if you read any of the books listed in the bibliography, you'll see just how sketchy and incomplete the information on liquid and gel soapmaking really is. What has been written is aimed at large-scale industrial soapmakers who already know the tricks of the trade. So, in addition to being an author, I've also had to function as a translator and an interpreter: translating industrial manufacturing techniques down to kitchen scale, and interpreting what seems to lie between the lines of those old soapmaking manuals. Which is just about everything.

This book has been a methodical labor of love, but I must confess that many discoveries happened quite by accident. I'm certain there's lots more out there to be learned and communicated about liquid soapmaking. I hope this book will offer a starting place for some other enterprising soul.

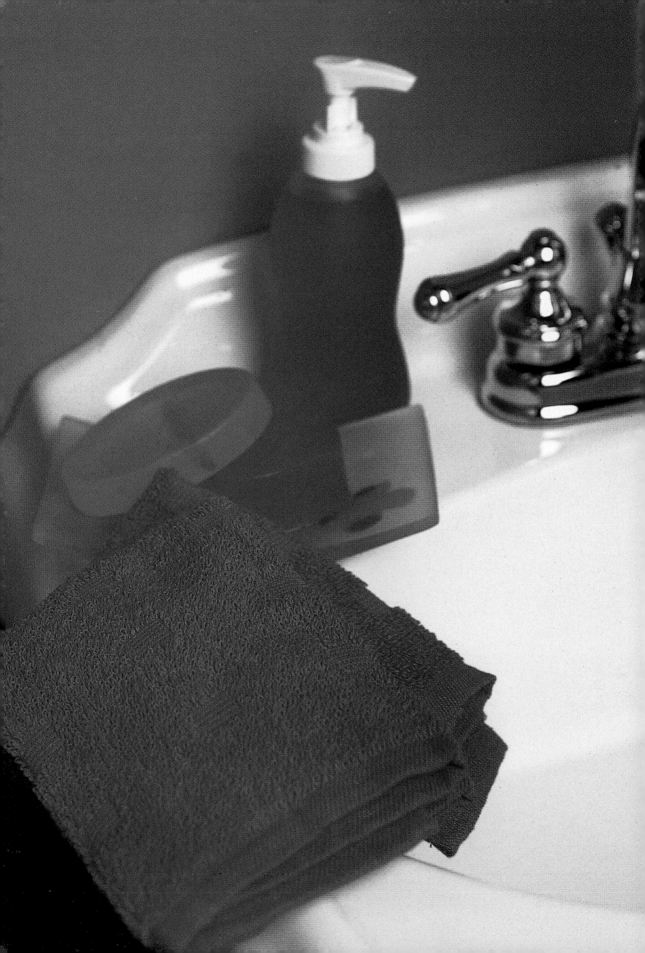

contents

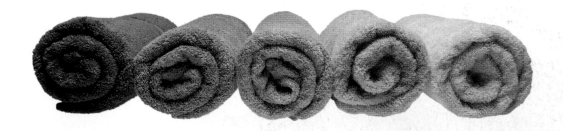

an introduction to soap

What is soap and how does it clean?

The words *soap* and *saponification* share the same etymological ancestor: *sapo,* the cleaning salve that the ancient Gauls prepared from animal fat mixed with wood ash. Modern chemistry has refined the raw materials as well as the technique, but soapmaking is basically the same as it was two thousand years ago: In a chemical reaction called saponification, a fatty acid (from either an animal or a vegetable source) combines with a solution of water and alkali (sodium or potassium hydroxide) to produce soap and glycerin.

It's All about the Chemistry

Oil and water, as the saying goes, don't mix. This presents a problem for soapmakers when a lye solution is added to fats, because all chemical reactions require that the two reactants be in contact. This difficulty is overcome by the chemical makeup of fats. Fats and oils are composed of triglycerides: three chainlike molecules of fatty acids attached to a single-molecule "spine" of glycerol in a configuration that loosely resembles the capital letter E. These triglycerides are tightly bonded molecules, but even the purest fats and oils always contain a small proportion of free fatty acids, or acid chains not attached to a glycerol molecule. When a caustic solution is added to a fat, saponification first takes place between these free fatty acids and the alkali. Small amounts of soap are formed.

Soap is an excellent emulsifier. The initial trace quantity of soap formed by the reaction between free fatty acids and alkali emulsifies unsaponified fat by breaking it up into small globules. The dispersed fat now has a much larger surface area that creates a larger "interface" between fat and alkali. Saponification proceeds more rapidly. (This principle has a very practical application for the home soapmaker: A few ounces of scrap soap, either sodium or potassium, can be dissolved in water, then used for making a lye solution. The soap emulsifies the fat, greatly reducing the stir time.)

When all available alkali has reacted with all available fatty acid, saponification is complete. Besides creating soap, this reaction yields glycerin, derived from the liberated glycerol molecule. Glycerin is typically "grained" (separated) out of commercial soap with common salt, then sold as a raw material. Glycerin remains in homemade soap, contributing emollient properties to the finished product.

Cleansing Action

Soap has a very contradictory nature. It has a water-loving, oil-hating "head," composed of sodium or potassium, and a water-hating, oil-loving "tail," consisting of a fatty acid chain. Soap's effectiveness as a cleaning agent stems directly from this contradiction, because soap acts as an intermediary between two very incompatible substances: oil and water.

Once soap has dissolved in water, the oil-loving parts of the soap molecules gravitate toward any patch of dirt on skin or fabric (a case of like attracting like) and form a ring around the soil called a *micelle*. These oil-loving tails break up the soil into smaller globules. Meanwhile, the water-loving halves of the molecules are straining outward toward the water in the sink or washing machine (again, like attracts like). The cleaning action of soap is thus a two-pronged process: a breaking up, as the oil-loving tails surround and emulsify soil, and a carrying away of soil, as the water-loving heads strain outward toward the surrounding water.

Sodium vs. Potassium Soaps

All true soaps, whether liquid or solid, are created through the reaction of an alkali with fatty acids. Sodium hydroxide and fatty acids produce hard bar soap through the crystallization of sodium. What you actually see when you look at a bar of soap is crystals; the bar appears opaque because the crystals cause light waves to bounce off the bar. Transparent bar soaps are also sodium-based, but they are see-through because the soap crystals have been largely dissolved in solvents such as alcohol, glycerin, and sugar. The light waves travel through the bar, making the soap appear transparent.

Potassium hydroxide is the base for all liquid soaps. Potassium is much more soluble than sodium and less able to form crystals. Liquid soaps are clear because light passes unobstructed through liquid soap much as it does through a bar of transparent soap.

Why Make Your Own Soap?

Before World War I, all liquid soaps were based on potassium hydroxide. But the shortage of fats and oils in wartime forced commercial soapmakers to consider other alternatives. Synthetic detergent soaps quickly became the norm and have remained so ever since. Many people today, though, are seeking alternatives to detergent soap, and potassium soap is ideal. It's formulated with pure, natural ingredients; can be tailored to fit different skin types; and is easy and inexpensive to make. Potassium soaps are also very versatile — one "base" formulation can be modified with just one or two ingredients to form a hand soap, a shampoo, or a bubble bath.

getting

① started

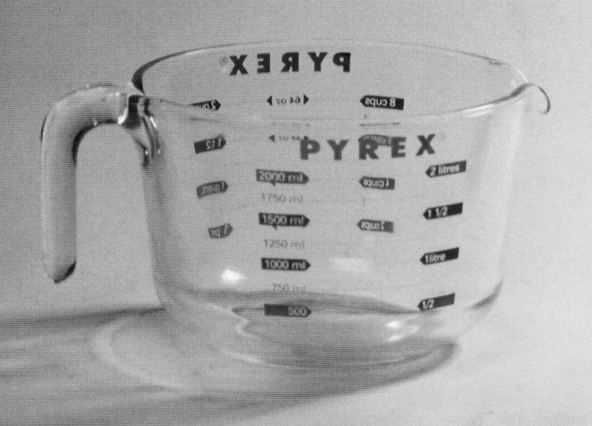

Water. Ammonium laureth sulfate. Glycol distearate. Cocamide MEA. Stearyl alcohol. Disodium EDTA. All very common liquid soap ingredients, but the only recognizable ingredient for most consumers is the water.

These laboratory-produced compounds are part of a long list of ingredients found in modern liquid soaps, which are actually detergents. Aside from their cleansing properties, these "soaps" have been engineered for stability because they're often shipped thousands of miles to market and suffer from exposure to heat, cold, and light. Before the days of international commerce and mass marketing, liquid soap was soap, often consisting of little else besides coconut oil and potassium hydroxide.

The ingredients and additives for "old-fashioned" liquid soap are listed in this chapter. You can formulate soap with a single oil and potassium hydroxide, or create blends of many oils enhanced with a wide variety of additives. A review of the procedures and recipes in the following chapters will help you decide before you spend your money.

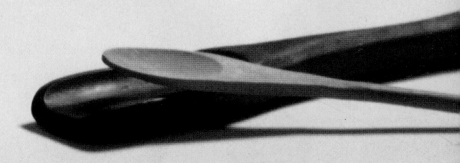

hard fats

Hard fats are composed primarily of stearic, palmitic, and lauric acids. These fatty acids are solid at room temperature, and the fats containing a predominance of these acids — whether tallow, coconut oil, or palm oil — also tend to be hard at room temperature.

Coconut Oil

Coconut oil forms the backbone of most liquid soap formulations. Why? Because of lauric acid, the predominant fatty acid in coconut oil. Lauric acid possesses one supreme virtue: solubility.

The more soluble the fatty acid, the less potential for cloudiness in the finished soap. Solubility also means that the soap has a quick, voluminous lather. This property is particularly important for liquid soaps because dilution by water reduces the soap's foaming action. The minerals contained in hard water also reduce lather, making coconut oil soaps the best performers in unsoftened water.

Because coconut oil–based liquid soaps are so soluble, higher proportions of soap to water are possible before the soap begins to congeal. A 100 percent coconut oil soap is still fluid at 40 percent soap to 60 percent water, whereas an olive oil soap begins to congeal at a much lower concentration: around 20 percent soap to 80 percent water. This is one reason why most public soap dispensers are filled with coconut-based liquid soap: This won't clog the dispenser.

One drawback of coconut oil is the drying effect of lauric acid. This negative property can be overcome by blending coconut oil with soft oils, such as olive, canola, or safflower oil. Palm kernel oil can be substituted for coconut oil because it has a similar fatty acid profile, but it requires approximately 20 percent less caustic than coconut oil for neutralization. See the chart on page 50 for specific information on the proportions of alkali to oils.

▶ A strong-bristle brush is a good tool for cleaning under fingernails with liquid hand soap.

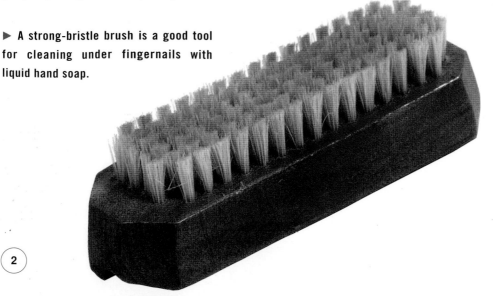

Palm Oil and Tallow

Palm oil and tallow possess characteristics that make them ideal bases for opaque hand soaps. They form rich, stable lathers and create a hard, long-lasting bar. These qualities are derived from the palmitic and stearic acids that constitute the bulk of both oils. But palmitic and stearic acids are mostly unwelcome in liquid soaps, where crystal clarity is desired. The two acids react with potassium hydroxide to form insoluble soaps, and these insolubles cloud an otherwise clear liquid. Used sparingly, however, palm oil or tallow gives extra "body" to liquid soap.

Cocoa Butter

Extracted from the roasted seeds of the cacao plant, cocoa butter is an excellent emollient and skin softener. Like palm oil and tallow, however, cocoa butter contains a high percentage of palmitic and stearic acids and should be used judiciously in liquid soap formulations.

> In gels, a small percentage of either palm oil or tallow helps prevent "thinning" of the gel during hot summer months.

▶ The base of liquid soap is potassium hydroxide, a water-soluble alkali.

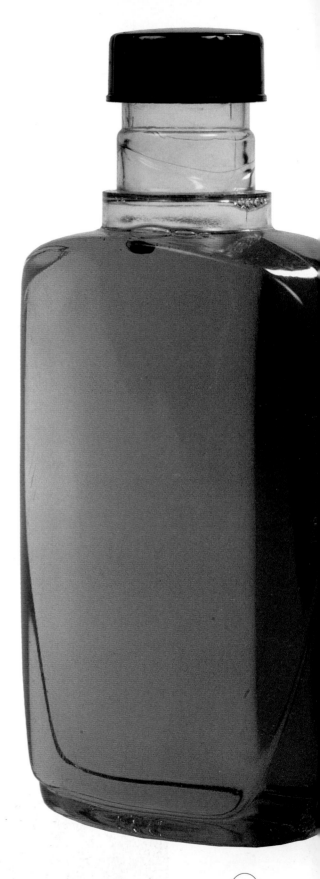

soft oils

Soft oils are generally liquid at room temperature: olive, canola, soybean, safflower, corn, or peanut oil. High in oleic, linoleic, and linolenic fatty acids, these oils form moisturizing soaps with thin, weak lathers. A mixture of 10 to 20 percent coconut oil and 80 to 90 percent soft oil forms a soap with enhanced foaming.

For liquid soap formulation, the choice of soft oils is up to the soapmaker because all soft oils (except castor oil) require a similar amount of alkali for neutralization. Aside from affordability and accessibility, these choices are in part aesthetic: How deeply colored is the oil? How strong is its odor? Dark oils, such as soybean oil, impart a markedly amber tone to liquid soap; strongly scented oils, such as sesame oil, can alter the fragrance of the finished soap.

Another consideration in the choice of oils is stability, or shelf life. Soft oils are unsaturated and therefore combine more readily with oxygen than saturated fats, such as coconut oil or tallow. Oxidation leads to rancidity. In general, oils high in linolenic acid are the least stable and most prone to rancidity (see the chart on the facing page). But this is a bit simplistic because many other factors influence the stability of a given oil, such as processing conditions, type of container, temperature of storage, and presence of natural antioxidants. It is safe to say that if you start with recently purchased oils that smell "clean" when opened, your finished soap should enjoy a long shelf life.

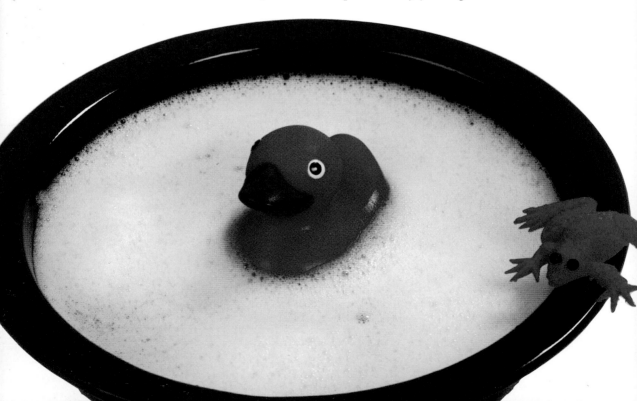

Important Fatty Acids in Common Fats and Oils

Fat or Oil	Percentage of Each Fatty Acid
Almond	69 oleic, 17 linoleic, 7 stearic
Avocado	62 oleic, 16 linoleic, 15 myristic, 6 palmitic
Babassu	44 lauric, 16 oleic, 15 myristic, 9 palmitic, 3 stearic, 2 linoleic
Canola	60 oleic, 22 linoleic, 10 linolenic, 4 palmitic, 2 stearic
Castor	87 ricinoleic, 7 oleic, 3 linoleic, 2 palmitic, 1 stearic
Cocoa butter	38 oleic, 35 stearic, 24 palmitic, 2 linoleic
Coconut	45 lauric, 20 myristic, 7 palmitic, 5 stearic, 4 oleic
Corn	50 oleic, 34 linoleic, 10 palmitic, 3 stearic
Lard	46 oleic, 28 palmitic, 13 stearic, 6 linoleic
Olive	85 oleic, 7 palmitic, 5 linoleic, 2 stearic
Palm	42 oleic, 40 palmitic, 10 linoleic, 5 stearic
Palm kernel	47 lauric, 19 oleic, 14 myristic, 9 palmitic, 1 stearic
Peanut	56 oleic, 26 linoleic, 8 palmitic, 3 stearic
Safflower	70 linoleic, 19 oleic
Sesame	41 linoleic, 39 oleic, 9 palmitic, 5 stearic
Soybean	51 linoleic, 29 oleic, 9 palmitic, 7 linolenic
Tallow	45 oleic, 28 palmitic, 25 stearic, 2 myristic
Wheat germ	52 linoleic, 28 oleic, 4 linoleic

 OTHER HIGH-OLEIC SOFT OILS

Canola, almond, corn, and peanut oils, like olive oil, are high-oleic soft oils. Avocado oil contains a high percentage of oleic acid but should be used sparingly because it also contains a fairly high percentage of substances that do not saponify and can cloud liquid soap.

Avoid formulating with vegetable shortening. Through the process of hydrogenation, unsaturated fatty acids are converted into their saturated analogs; for example, unsaturated oleic acid becomes saturated stearic acid. Saturated acids form insoluble soaps, which consequently produce milky liquids.

◄ A combination of coconut oil and soft oils will produce the most successful liquid soap.

Olive Oil

Olive oil, which is 85 percent oleic acid, has been the favorite of soapmakers for centuries. It penetrates the skin better than almost any other vegetable oil except castor oil. The resulting soaps are moisturizing as well as mild, making olive oil an excellent base for baby shampoo.

Castor Oil

Castor oil is in a class of its own. It's part oil and part alcohol — a peculiarity derived from the molecular structure of ricinoleic acid, the fatty acid accounting for almost 90 percent of castor oil's bulk. Alcohols act as solvents, and castor oil's solvency is readily apparent in soapmaking; it speeds saponification and adds exceptional clarity to both transparent and liquid soaps. This explains why castor oil is the only soft oil you'll ever see in transparent bar formulations. Aside from its transparency-producing virtues, castor oil is exceptionally mild and is easily absorbed by the skin, making it an excellent emollient and moisturizer.

Soapmaking Properties of Common Fats and Oils

Fat or Oil	Lather Characteristics	Cleaning Properties	Action on Skin	Appearance in Liquid Soap	How Saponified
Almond	oily, close, persistent	fair to good	very mild	clear	fairly easily
Canola	oily, close, medium-lasting	fair	mild	clear	fairly easily
Castor	thick, lasting	fair	mild	very clear	very easily
Coconut	quick, foamy bubbles, does not persist	excellent	biting action, roughens skin	clear	quickly
Olive	oily, close, persistent	fair to good	very mild	clear	fairly easily
Palm	slow, lasting, close	very good	very mild	very cloudy	very easily
Palm kernel	quick, foamy large bubbles, doesn't persist	excellent	biting action, roughens skin	clear	quickly
Rosin	oily, thick	fair	mild	very clear	very quickly
Soybean	oily, abundant, medium-lasting	fair	mild	clear	fairly easily
Tallow	fairly slow, lasting, thick	good	very mild	very cloudy	fairly easily

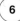

Sulfonated Castor Oil

Also known as "turkey red oil," sulfonated castor oil is created by the reaction between castor oil and sulfuric acid. This oil first proved useful to the textile industry over a century ago; its water-soluble nature not only allowed for better penetration of dyes into wool and other fabrics but also increased the brightness and luster of the colors. "Turkey red" refers to the brilliant red color produced specifically on cotton cloth.

Water solubility makes sulfonated castor oil an ideal superfatting agent in liquid soapmaking, adding the lubricity of an oil without compromising the clarity of the soap. Sulfonated castor oil forms the base of "soapless" shampoos (see recipe in chapter 4) and is effective in both hard and soft water. As an unsaponifiable oil, it should never be substituted for regular castor oil in soap formulations.

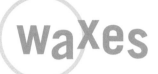

Waxes

Waxes are chemically similar to oils except that the wax molecules are composed of more alcohol than glycerol. Small additions of a wax to liquid soaps enhance the moisturizing properties of the lather.

Lanolin

Lanolin, produced from the oil glands of sheep, is a water-absorbent base material and consequently an effective moisturizer. Because lanolin contains a high percentage of substances that do not saponify, it clouds liquid soap and should be limited to 1 to 2 percent of any formulation.

Jojoba

Jojoba, which is similar to the sebum produced by our own oil glands, is a liquid wax derived from the seeds of a desert shrub. Mexicans and Native Americans have long used the oil as a hair conditioner and skin moisturizer; modern marketers promote its usefulness as a sunscreen and treatment for wrinkles, crow's feet, and dry skin. Like lanolin, it contains substances that do not saponify, and it must be used sparingly if crystal-clear soaps are desired.

potassium hydroxide (caustic potash)

Because of its solubility, potassium hydroxide forms the ideal base for all liquid soaps. Manufactured commercially from the electrolysis of potassium chloride, potassium hydroxide is sold as a liquid or crystalline flake. It's much more chemically reactive than sodium hydroxide, and more potassium than sodium hydroxide is needed to saponify a given amount of fat — 1.4 times more, to be precise.

solvents

The solvents alcohol, glycerin, and sugar are what enable a soapmaker to transform opaque bar soap into transparent soap. The solvents literally dissolve the soap crystals and then hold them in suspension, allowing the light to pass through.

Solvents are very useful in liquid soapmaking. The soap can be dissolved and "cooked" in alcohol (see The Alcohol/Lye Method on page 33), and small additions of alcohol, glycerin, and sugar will improve the brightness and clarity of the finished liquid.

Alcohol

Alcohols are solvents. In liquid soapmaking, solvents can speed saponification as well as lower a liquid's "cloud point," or the point at which insoluble substances precipitate out of solution. When liquid soaps are slightly cloudy because of excess fatty acids or minerals, a small addition of alcohol often clarifies the solution. Excess alcohol, however, reduces the sudsing action of the soap.

The liquid soapmaker has a choice of two types of alcohol: ethanol or isopropyl alcohol.

▶ Alcohol, glycerin, and sugar lower the cloud point of liquid soap, helping create crystal clarity.

Ethanol. Colorless and odorless, ethanol is produced from the fermentation of sugar, starch, and other carbohydrates. In liquor stores, ethanol is sold under the brand names Everclear and Clear Springs. Scientific supply houses sell denatured ethanol in gallon containers — a much cheaper option than pure liquor store ethanol. When ordering denatured alcohol, be sure to specify SDA (specially denatured alcohol) 3A or SDA 3C, two cosmetic grades approved by the FDA. Both have been denatured with trace amounts of isopropyl alcohol and methanol.

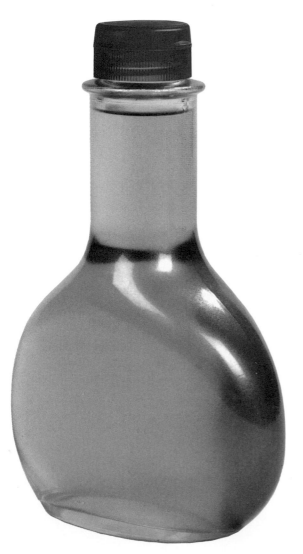

Isopropyl alcohol. Common isopropyl alcohol, or rubbing alcohol, can also be used for liquid soapmaking. As a solvent, it's "weaker" than ethanol, but because potassium soaps are so soluble, this weakness isn't a handicap. The strong odor of isopropyl alcohol can potentially taint the finished liquid, but this problem is easily rectified by evaporating the alcohol out of solution at the end of the soapmaking process.

All drugstores carry isopropyl alcohol, usually at a 70 percent strength (the remaining 30 percent is water). For the purposes of liquid soapmaking, stronger concentrations, in the range of 90 to 99 percent, are desirable. Many pharmacies stock the stronger solutions on the shelf, and some will special-order 99 percent concentrations; otherwise, contact the nearest scientific supply house.

Glycerin

A natural by-product of saponification, glycerin is technically an alcohol. Added to finished liquid soap, it lowers the cloud point the same way alcohol does, helping clarify residual milkiness. In addition, it functions as a humectant, drawing moisture from the air and holding it to the skin. Like ethanol or isopropyl alcohol, excessive amounts of glycerin dampen the foaming action of soap, though small amounts actually boost the foam. Purchase glycerin at pharmacies or through the suppliers listed in Resources.

other key ingredients

In the strictest sense, soap consists of a hydroxide in chemical combination with a fat. But many other ingredients determine the appearance and quality of the finished soap — what kind of water is used for both the lye solution and the dilution of the soap base, how the soap is thickened and preserved, and what to use for creating a neutral pH. The following are descriptions of some of these ingredients.

Sugar

Small percentages of sugar solution added to liquid soaps help dissipate cloudiness. Ounce for ounce, sugar is a more effective clarifier than glycerin, though it lacks glycerin's moisturizing properties.

Soft or Distilled Water

Minerals in hard water react with fatty acids to form insoluble fatty acid salts. The result? Cloudiness, much like the cloudiness formed by insoluble palmitic and stearic acid soaps mentioned earlier. For this reason, the use of soft or distilled water is essential for all phases of liquid soap production.

Rosin

Pears, the very first transparent soap, was formulated with rosin. Distilled from the oleoresin of pine trees, rosin saponifies much like an oil, but without any resulting glycerin. It imparts clarity to soap and a smooth cold-cream finish to the lather. It also acts as a detergent and preservative. Sold as fragrant, amber-colored crystals, rosin can be purchased through the suppliers listed in Resources.

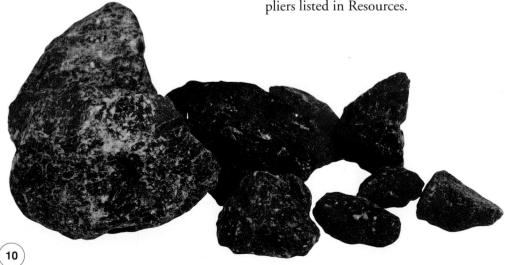

Borax, or Sodium Borate

The detergent and water-softening properties of borax were first discovered by Native Americans, who noticed that clothing washed in streams near borax deposits came out cleaner.

Borax is one of the best all-around additives for liquid soaps, possessing many desirable qualities. It's a viscosity modifier (thickener), an emulsifier, a water softener, a moisturizer, a foam booster and stabilizer, a pH buffer, and a preservative. Pharmacies carry borax (often behind the counter, so ask if it's not on the shelf), or it can be obtained from the suppliers listed in Resources.

Calgon

Like borax, Calgon brand bath preparation enhances foaming, softens hard water, and triggers gelling in liquid soaps. Calgon is a blend of various sodium salts, mainly sodium carbonate and sodium hexametaphosphate. Buy the "nonfoaming bath" variety. One drawback of Calgon is that the finished soap turns blue because of the dye in the powder.

◄ **Rosin, which is readily available from soapmaking suppliers, enhances the clarity and texture of liquid soap.**

Neutralizers

The recipes in this book all contain slight excesses of potassium hydroxide. This ensures that no unneutralized fatty acids remain at the end of saponification. The excess alkali can be neutralized with an acid. Boric acid, the buffer of choice used by old-time liquid soapmakers, can be found in any pharmacy. Citric acid also works. Wine-making supply shops carry citric acid, or it can be purchased through the suppliers listed in Resources.

Borax, at a pH of 9.2, is also an excellent neutralizer. If you use borax as a thickener in any formulation, no additional neutralizers will be necessary.

Potassium Carbonate

Potassium soap bases are quite sticky and viscous; stirring them is almost as difficult as stirring hot tar. One additive used by old-time liquid soapmakers to loosen the soap was potassium carbonate, or pearl ash. Pearl ash is a salt of potassium. When it is added to a potassium paste, the molecules of the carbonate actually insert themselves between the molecules of potassium hydroxide, making the soap much more pliable. Potassium carbonate is an optional ingredient, but if you'd like to experiment with it, purchase it through any scientific supply house.

Preservatives

The most effective preservative for liquid soap is complete saponification. Oxygenated fats trigger rancidity. Because oxygen attaches most readily to free fatty acids, it follows that thoroughly neutralized soap offers no oxidation sites. Fresh, clean-smelling soft oils are also very important because soft oils are by their very nature unsaturated and are more receptive to oxygen than saturated fats such as coconut oil and palm oil. A completely saponified rancid oil will produce a rancid-smelling soap. No amount of cooking reverses preexisting rancidity.

Many additives in liquid soap — such as borax, glycerin, alcohol, rosin, and citric acid — also act as preservatives. Certain essential oils, such as clary sage, also have preservative properties.

If you wish to use preservatives, use a mixed-tocopherol vitamin E. Vitamin E is composed of many types of tocopherols, such as alpha, gamma, and omega. The alpha tocopherols are effective for healing skin but not for preserving soaps. If you specifically purchase mixed-tocopherol vitamin E, you're getting the optimum preservative in vitamin E form.

Another new product on the market is rosemary extract, an excellent antioxidant. Some of the suppliers listed in Resources carry rosemary extract.

Many soapmakers use grapefruit seed oil for its supposed preservative properties, but grapefruit seed oil functions as an antifungal and antibacterial agent, not as an antioxidant.

Biocides

Does liquid soap need an antibacterial agent, such as grapefruit seed extract or its commercial derivative, Citricidal? Many people assume that it does, but this assumption is based on the chemistry of the synthetic soaps that now predominate the market. These soaps typically fall within a pH range of 6 to 7, close to the neutral pH of water. Neutral pHs are microbe-friendly; synthetic soaps are consequently bolstered with plenty of antimicrobial chemicals.

True soap doesn't suffer from this problem because it possesses a pH hostile to microbial growth. Bacteria shun alkaline environments above a pH of 9; neutral potassium soaps fall within a pH range of 9.5 to 10. Unless your soap is overacidified with a neutralizer such as citric acid, you needn't worry about bacteria growing in your homemade liquid soap.

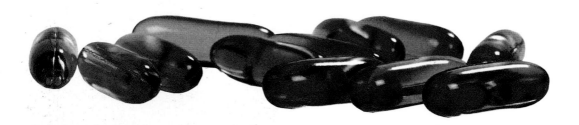

phenolphthalein

No text on hot-process soapmaking would be complete without mentioning this important chemical. Phenolphthalein (pronounced fee-nol-THA-leen) is a quirky chemical with diverse applications. It's found in laxatives and is a component of dyes.

For the soapmaker, phenolphthalein works as an acid-base indicator, turning pink to red in the presence of excess alkali and remaining clear in the presence of excess fatty acids. Many home soapmakers use pH strips to determine their soap's alkalinity/acidity, but these strips are basically worthless. Their subtle color gradations are almost impossible to read, and even if a reading is "approximately" correct, approximate isn't always enough for liquid soap.

Phenolphthalein can be purchased either in a liquid form or as a powder, which is then diluted in alcohol. Buy it through any of the suppliers listed in Resources, or call a scientific supply house.

◄ Vitamin E is an antioxidant that can help extend the shelf life of homemade soap.

► Display your creations in unusual or fun bottles!

Phenolphthalein isn't on the "required ingredient" list, but diagnosing and correcting problem soap become very difficult without it. See the box on page 14 for complete instructions on using phenolphthalein.

Home soapmakers often spend hundreds of dollars on tools such as scales, thermometers, and mixers. Consider a small, inexpensive bottle of phenolphthalein to be an equally important tool.

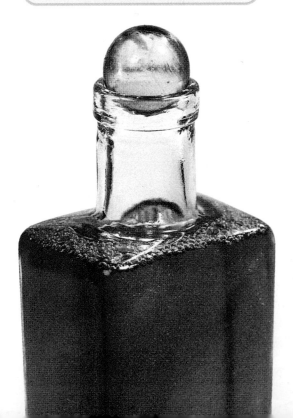

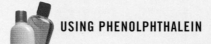

USING PHENOLPHTHALEIN

To prepare a test solution, add a few drops of phenolphthalein to a pound of ethanol or isopropyl alcohol. Then stir in a very small amount of weak potassium hydroxide solution; add until a faint pink color develops in the alcohol. When testing soap, an ounce or two of this test solution is all that's needed.

Determine the alkalinity or acidity of the soap by removing a sample spoonful of finished paste or alcohol broth. Do this before diluting the entire batch with water. If the pH needs correcting, it's much easier to work with undiluted soap because oils and alkalis can't adequately react when diluted with large amounts of water.

To prepare a sample, dissolve 1 ounce of soap paste or alcohol broth in 2 ounces of hot water. Stir the dissolved soap into 1 to 2 ounces of phenolphthalein test solution. The soap contains excess alkali if the test solution turns a deeper shade of pink. The deeper the color, the more alkaline the soap. Some pink color should be expected because the recipes in this book are all slightly overalkalized. By adding 8 to 12 drops of 20 percent citric or boric acid solution to the phenolphthalein test sample, the solution should turn a faint pink to clear, indicating neutrality. If the test solution remains a strong pink, you can correct the pH using the technique outlined in chapter 8 for overalkaline soap.

If the test solution becomes clear with the addition of soap solution, the soap contains excess fatty acids. This isn't necessarily a problem. Determine whether it's a problem by dissolving another ounce of paste or broth in hot water. Allow the sample to cool. If it remains clear upon cooling, then the excess fatty acids aren't detrimental — in fact, they'll add extra emollience. If the solution clouds, then correct the problem using the technique outlined in chapter 8 for excess fatty acids.

Note: If phenolphthalein is added to neutral soap stock, the soap will turn pink when mixed with tap water. This is caused not by excess alkalinity but by hydrolysis, the splitting up of the soap molecule by water into fatty acids and alkali. Liberated alkalis react with the phenolphthalein; hence, the pink color.

basic equipment

Before pulling out your wallet and heading for the store, look in your kitchen and workshop for the equipment listed here. You'll probably be able to find (or borrow) almost everything on this list. Have you already made cold-process soap? If so, a candy thermometer may be your only new expense.

Thermometer

Another, equally important piece of equipment is an accurate candy or deep-fry thermometer capable of measuring up to 160 to 170°F (71 to 76°C). Most grocery stores and specialty kitchen shops carry these thermometers; make sure yours has a stainless steel stem.

Scale

An accurate scale is the most important (as well as expensive) investment you'll have to make. It must indicate 1-ounce increments and have a minimum capacity of 10 pounds. For used, reconditioned equipment, look under Scales in the Yellow Pages.

Cooking Pot

An 8- to 12-quart enamel or stainless steel cooking pot will function as your soap pot. Make sure it is enamel or stainless steel, because alkalis corrode other metals, particularly aluminum.

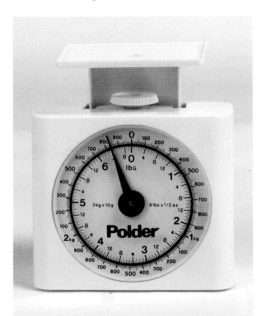

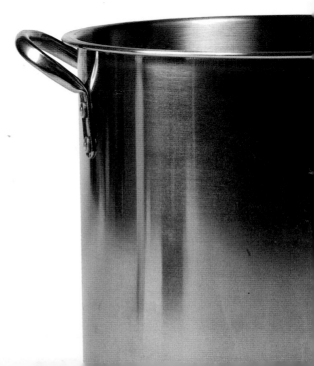

5-Gallon Canning Pot

Hot processing is done in a double boiler; this is the closest a home soapmaker can come to the steam kettles used in commercial soapmaking. Your 8- to 12-quart soap pot will be placed in a larger kettle partially filled with boiling water. This keeps the temperature constant (soap cooked in this manner will not get so hot that it "erupts") and prevents the soap from scorching. A 5-gallon canning pot is ideal. Whatever you use, make certain your soap pot fits completely inside the larger kettle. (This second pot needn't be enamel or stainless steel, because no caustic soap comes in contact with it.) If you don't already own one, 5-gallon kettles are relatively easy to find at secondhand shops and garage sales.

Stirrers and Mixers

If you're hand-stirring soap, stainless steel whisks work better than spoons because they're better at emulsifying the oil-lye solution. The faster a solution is emulsified, the quicker the rate of saponification.

Many home soapmakers rely on stick blenders, regular upright blenders, or food processors for the tracing phase of soapmaking. This rapid mechanical motion speeds saponification by speeding the emulsification of oil and lye. Some formulations will trace within 5 to 10 minutes; by contrast, hand-mixing can require 30 to 60 minutes of constant stirring before the soap traces. With a stick blender, no caustic soap solutions need to be transferred from one container to another, and cleanup is also much simpler.

◄ **Make a double boiler by placing your soap pot inside a canning pot.**

▼ **Metal whisks and metal or wooden spoons are all suitable for soapmaking.**

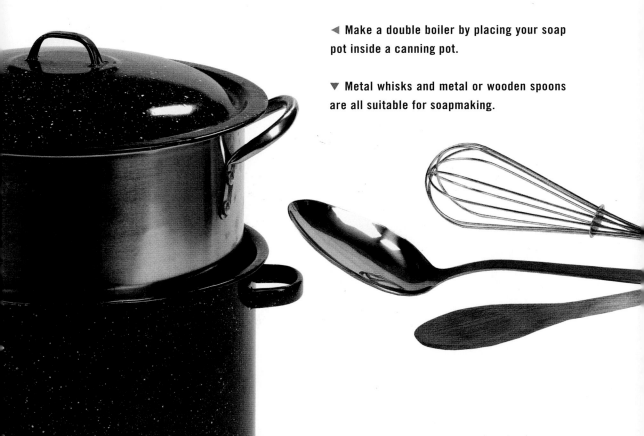

Goggles and Gloves

Unneutralized soap is extremely caustic, and care must be taken to protect the skin and eyes. Always wear goggles and gloves, particularly before the soap has completely neutralized.

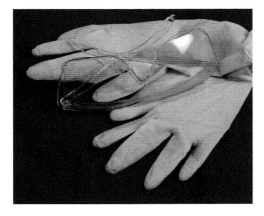

Sheeting and Bungee Cords

If you follow the alcohol-lye method outlined in the following chapter, you'll need plastic sheeting and two bungee cords. The plastic will be stretched over the top of your cooking pot and fastened with bungee cords, ensuring that the alcohol in solution isn't lost to evaporation.

Buy 3- or 4-ml clear plastic, which allows you to view the cooking soap. This thick-gauge plastic can be found in any hardware or paint supply store. Thick plastic is very important because it must be able to stretch without breaking as the alcohol and steam expand in the soap pot. For this reason, don't use Saran Wrap or any other thin kitchen plastic wrap.

Bottles and Jars

One advantage of liquid soapmaking is that the soap base can be refrigerated indefinitely until you're ready to dilute it down into a liquid or gel. At that point, you'll need containers. Start now to collect containers around your home, or visit secondhand shops. Bottle suppliers are listed in Resources.

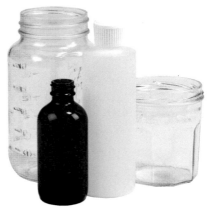

▲ Glass and plastic are both appropriate materials for containers.

▼ Plastic sheeting and bungee cords are available at most hardware stores.

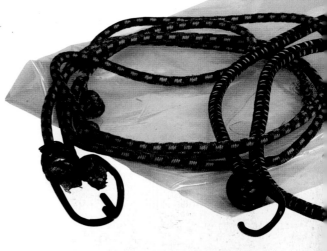

a guide ② to basic techniques

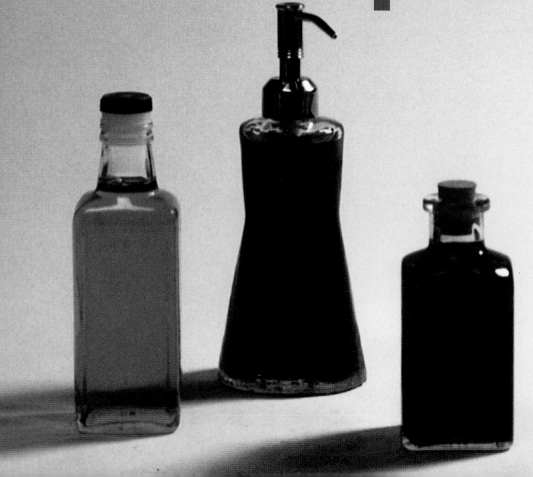

old-process soap has been the queen of the kitchen for almost 30 years, since the publication of Ann Bramson's *Soap: Making It, Enjoying It.* The procedures for cold processing are now so familiar that some soapmakers jest that they can make soap blindfolded, with one hand tied behind their backs!

Hot processing is new and unfamiliar, and unfamiliarity breeds uncertainty and reluctance. But the hot-processing procedure is actually very simple, and with just a little experience it all becomes second nature. Even better, all soaps currently on the market can now be made in your kitchen.

For small soap businesses there's an extra incentive: Liquid and gel soaps now account for approximately 25 percent of annual soap sales in the U.S., but small-scale soapmakers have yet to create a presence in this market.

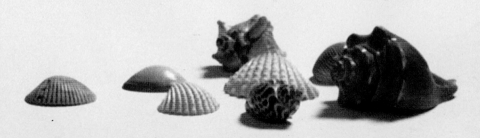

hot-process soapmaking

Why hot-process? Because it offers two things everyone loves: control and variety.

Hot processing is a simple technique whereby a soap base is cooked at relatively high temperatures (180–200°F; 82–93°C) for 2 to 3 hours. Elevated temperatures ensure that all the free fatty acids are neutralized, which is critical for producing crystal-clear liquid soaps and transparent bar soaps. Hot processing is necessary for producing other specialty soaps — such as floating soap, creams and pastes, and translucent bars — as well. And if mistakes are made, most of them are correctable. This is why hot processing has been the method of choice for commercial soapmakers throughout the centuries.

Cold processing, by contrast, involves no cooking of the soap base. Oils and lye solution are combined at relatively low temperatures (80–100°F; 26–38°C), and then the emulsion is poured into molds, insulated with blankets, and left alone for approximately 24 hours. During this time the soap is cooking itself, heated by the reaction between the fatty acids and the alkali.

Most home soapmaking is done by the cold-process method, but cold processing has many limitations. It's a one-trick pony that produces lovely opaque hand soaps, but that's about it. Clear liquids and bars, creams, and floating soaps are all beyond the technique's scope. In addition, once the soap is poured into the molds, "cross your fingers and hope" is a familiar scenario with many cold-process soapmakers. Cross your fingers and hope that what appears the next day is soap, not soup. The cold-process technique offers one chance to get things right; soap made from mismeasured ingredients or temperature is usually punished with a trip to the trash can.

Here I present two methods for hot processing soap. Derived from techniques first introduced in my book *Making Transparent Soap,* each method has its own personality, interest, and appeal. Study both methods, then select a recipe from chapter 3. Make the recipe according to both methods; this will help you decide which technique you prefer.

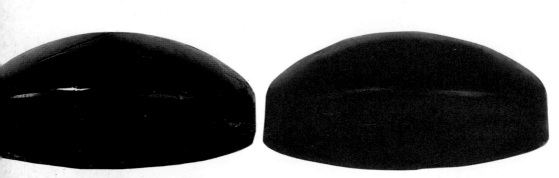

the golden rule

If there's one basic liquid soapmaking principle that needs to be underlined, emphasized, and shouted from the rooftops, it's this: *Unneutralized fatty acids cause cloudiness.*

When a caustic solution of either sodium or potassium hydroxide is added to fat, the fatty acids separate from the glycerol in a process called hydrolysis (from the Greek *hydro*, meaning "water," and *lysis*, "setting free"). Hydrolysis is a form of decomposition. These liberated fatty acids then combine chemically with the sodium or potassium ions to form soap. If an insufficient amount of alkali has been added, if excess oils are present, or if the temperature of the saponifying soap stock is relatively low, unneutralized fatty acids remain in the soap. For opaque hand soaps, these fatty acids can be most desirable, adding extra richness and emollience to the lather. Home soapmakers capitalize on these qualities by purposefully "superfatting" their soaps.

▶ **Hot processing is the only method that produces truly clear soap, whether in bars or liquid form.**

Achieving Transparency

Excess fatty acids are disastrous in transparent bars, liquids, or gels. This excess manifests as an opaque milkiness. If you've ever attempted to make a clear soap using the cold-process method, you've undoubtedly met with failure because no matter how accurately you measure your oils and alkalis, the process seldom generates enough heat to completely neutralize the fatty acids.

Saponification is a heat-generating chemical reaction. Within reason, the more heat, the more complete the reaction. Hot processing adds the mechanical heat from your kitchen stove to the chemical heat created through saponification. Added heat bonds all the available fatty acids with the alkali. The result? Clear, neutral soap.

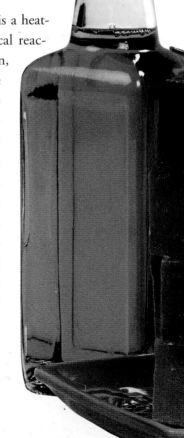

the paste method

The paste method bears some resemblance to cold-process soapmaking. A caustic solution is added to warm fats, then stirred until the mixture thickens, or traces. But the hot and cold processes diverge here; in hot processing, traced soap is further cooked in a double boiler until neutral.

1 Prepare the Double Boiler

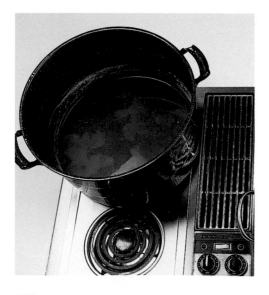

Fill a 5-gallon canning pot (or any pot large enough to contain the soap pot) with 3 or 4 inches of water. This will become the bottom of the double boiler. Place it on a back burner, cover it, and begin heating the water. You'll want a gentle boil for cooking soap.

2 Add the Fats and Oils

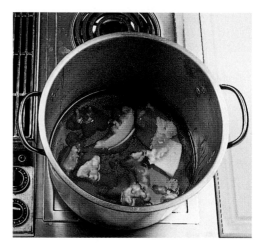

To prepare the fats, first weigh the fats and oils, then empty them into the soap pot, and place this pot over medium heat. Melt any hard fats or waxes first, then add soft oils. Continue heating until the oils reach 160°F (71°C). Turn the heat to low, and maintain this temperature.

> The temperature of a potassium solution is considerably lower than that of a pure sodium solution because it has roughly 50 percent more water. The extra water "quenches" some of the reaction's heat.

3 Prepare a Lye Solution

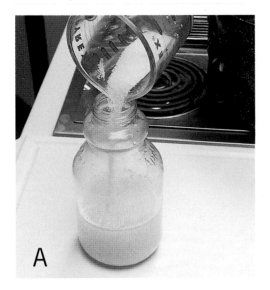

A

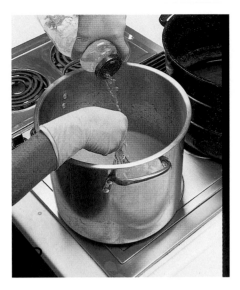

Put on your goggles and gloves, measure out the water portion of the solution, and pour it into a 2-quart (or larger) glass, ceramic, stainless steel, or heavy plastic container.

➲ Weigh the potassium hydroxide.

➲ **Add the flakes to the water (A), and stir until dissolved (B).** Be careful to avoid inhaling the steam that's given off: The temperature will rise to 150°F (65°C) almost instantly, and the steam itself is slightly caustic.

➲ If you're adding potassium carbonate (pearl ash) to the soap, now is the time to mix it in. Stir the powdered carbonate into the hot lye solution to ensure that the carbonate dissolves completely.

 WARNING: POTASSIUM HYDROXIDE

Potassium hydroxide is quite caustic and can cause chemical burns on contact. Always use goggles and gloves when handling raw flakes, lye solutions, and unneutralized soap. Store these substances in well-sealed, breakproof, clearly labeled containers away from children and pets. In case of contact with skin or eyes, rinse for several minutes with water. Lemon juice or vinegar is also effective for instantly neutralizing hydroxide on the skin, but don't splash these acids in eyes. In case of ingestion, call the local poison control center.

4 Add the Lye to the Oils

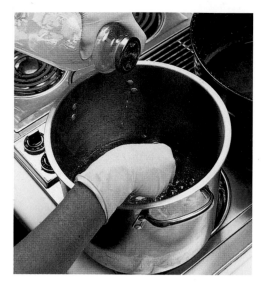

5 Stir

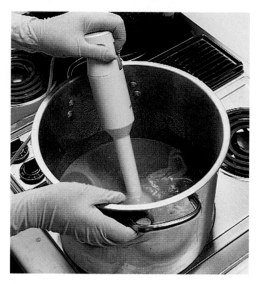

Allow the caustic solution to cool to approximately 140°F (60°C). **In a slow, steady stream, add the solution to the 160°F (71°C) oils, stirring constantly.** One way to obtain a slow, consistent flow is to mix the caustic flakes and water in a 2-quart jar fitted with a metal lid. Before mixing the water and flakes, punch two holes in the lid with an ice pick or screwdriver. The two holes should be opposite each other (12 o'clock and 6 o'clock), and one hole should be larger than the other. The solution will be poured from the larger hole; the smaller hole simply allows air into the jar.

Stir with a whisk or stick blender. If you have any experience with sodium-based soaps, potassium soapmaking may initially perplex you. The stir phase for sodium soap follows a gradual and predictable curve from thin to thick. Potassium soap stock can remain stubbornly thin for some time before suddenly thickening. It's very important to stir until the soap becomes quite viscous; otherwise, separation may occur between the potassium solution and the soap stock. In addition, the more thorough the mixing, the more thorough the saponification.

> Make sure to stir the oil and lye solution in the soap pot before adding it to the blender; the oil and lye separate easily when left sitting.

Don't stop stirring at these first signs of thickening. Within a few minutes, the thickened stock further changes to the consistency of sticky, saltwater taffy. The more coconut oil in the formulation, the stickier the mass. Formulations high in soft oils won't initially be quite as sticky; it takes an hour or so of cooking for soft oils to reach a taffylike consistency. This is because soft oils aren't as soluble as coconut oil.

The time needed to reach this phase depends on several factors: the temperature of the stock, the oil type, and your stir speed. Throughout the stirring, maintain a temperature of 160 to 170°F (71 to 76°C). Heat accelerates the saponification rate. Because of differences in chemical makeup, some oils saponify more readily than others. Coconut and castor oil, for example, react with an alkali much more rapidly than olive oil. And hand-stirring is to stick-blending what the tortoise is to the hare.

Here are a few tips to help you economize stir time:

➲ If you choose to hand-stir, a whisk mixes more efficiently than a spoon or spatula because it speeds emulsification of the oils and lye.

➲ A stick blender is more flexible, versatile, and tidy than a traditional blender or food processor, but all three tools cut an extraordinary amount of time out of stirring. If you are using a blender or food processor, fill the vessels only about half full to allow headroom for any "puffing up" of the thickening soap as air is incorporated. Always keep the cap on the blender when mixing.

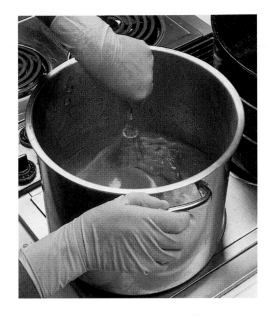

➲ **Mix the hot oils and the lye the night before, stirring for just 5 or 10 minutes.** Cover the soap pot with a blanket or two to conserve heat, then let it stand overnight. During this time small amounts of soap will form, serving as a "starter" by lowering the surface tension between lye and oils. The next day, heat the mixture back up to 160 to 170°F (71 to 76°C) and stir until thickened.

A variation on the "starter" method above:

After making your first batch of soap, set aside 3 or 4 ounces of neutral, undiluted paste, then refrigerate it in a jar or plastic bag until your next round of soapmaking. Add this paste to the oil and lye solution, taking care to mix and dissolve it thoroughly. You'll be amazed at how much time it trims off stirring.

➲ A few ounces of alcohol, either ethanol or isopropyl alcohol, added to the oil and lye solution will speed saponification by lowering the surface tension between the oil/lye interface.

6 Cook the Paste

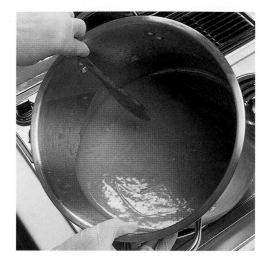

Check to make sure that the soap has thickened. Then place the soap pot into the gently boiling water of the double boiler bottom. If the larger pot has a lid, use it; this will both conserve heat and keep your kitchen from steaming up. The total cooking time for the paste will be 3 hours.

➲ After 5 or 10 minutes of cooking, remove the soap pot from the double boiler bottom, and check for lye separation. Potassium solutions will separate from the paste if the paste was under-stirred. If separation has occurred, it appears as a watery layer at the bottom of the pot. Stir again — it won't take long to incorporate this solution back into the paste. Then set the pot back into the kettle and continue cooking. In another 5 or 10 minutes, check for separation one more time. Stir again if necessary.

➲ Don't be alarmed if the paste puffs up. Potassium pastes are so sticky that they readily trap air in the initial stir phase. During cooking, this air heats and expands, creating a "soufflé" effect. A few stirs with a spoon or spatula allow the air to escape. If left in the soap, trapped air actually slows the saponification rate. You may need to stir another time or two over the next half hour to liberate all the trapped air, but the puffing eventually subsides. If the paste continues to puff up after an hour or more of cooking, you may have a problem with excess alkali. Consult chapter 8.

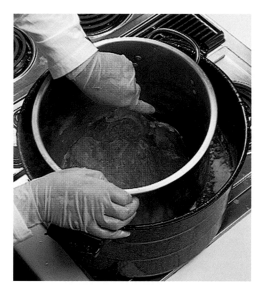

➲ **Stir the paste for a few minutes every 20 or 30 minutes over the next 3 hours.** During this time, you'll notice a change in the paste's appearance. Initially, it's opaque and off-white; after an hour or so, it gradually becomes translucent. This is a sign that the soap is neutralizing. If the paste shows no signs of translucence after 2 hours, the problem may be excess alkalinity. See chapter 8 for more information.

7 Test for Excess Fatty Acids

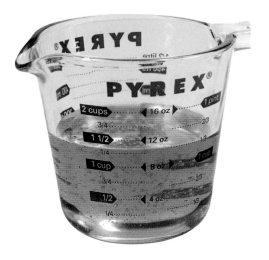

At the end of the 3-hour cook time, look for signs of free fatty acids by dissolving 1 ounce of soap in 2 ounces of boiling distilled water. The hot liquid may be clear, but the real determinant of thoroughly cooked soap is the appearance of the solution after it's cooled down. A cool sample will be slightly cloudy because of the presence of insoluble soaps, but these soaps will eventually settle out of solution. You can read more about insoluble soaps on page 109.

➲ A cooled sample that exhibits a pronounced milkiness indicates that the paste still contains unneutralized free fatty acids and needs more cooking and stirring. Return the soap to the double boiler and cook some more. After another 30 minutes, test again. If the soap doesn't test clearer after 4 hours of cooking, you've probably mismeasured the ingredients. Consult chapter 8 for help. Learning to discern the difference between normal clouding that will clear upon sequestering (described on page 31) and clouding that's a permanent problem is a matter of some experience. Rest assured that if you measure ingredients correctly and cook for the proper length of time, your soap will clear after sequestering.

> Always either use soft or distilled water in your liquid soap recipes. The minerals in hard water combine chemically with fatty acids, marring the transparency of the finished soap.

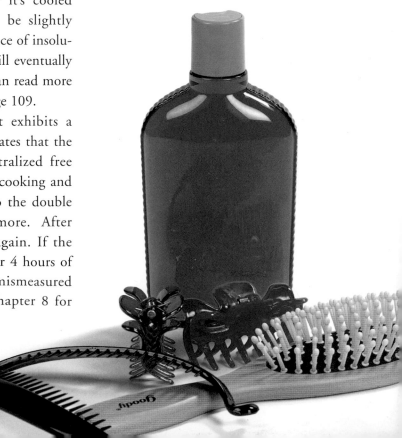

8 Dilute the Soap

After testing for free fatty acids, the soap is ready for dilution. A chart on soap-to-water dilution ratios appears on page 42. If you wish to dilute your soap later, or save a portion of the paste for a "starter" for your next batch, spoon the paste into a plastic bag and store in the refrigerator. The soap can be kept indefinitely in this manner, as refrigeration prevents the development of any possible rancidity.

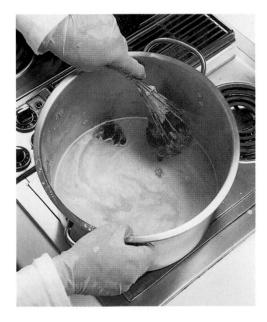

➲ **Bring the water to a boil, then add the paste; use a whisk or spoon to help break the mass up.** Pastes high in coconut oil dissolve more readily than those high in soft oils. If you desire a highly concentrated soap solution, be aware that the stronger the concentration, the more resistant the paste is to dissolving.

USING POTASSIUM CARBONATE

Other than dissolving the paste in alcohol, potassium carbonate is the only way to make potassium soap softer and more stirrable. Add potassium carbonate at a rate of 2 to 2.5 percent of the total weight of paste. As each recipe in this book yields approximately 6 pounds of paste, or about 100 ounces, add up to 2 or 2.5 ounces of dry pearl ash per recipe. The powder should be stirred into the hot lye solution.

Potassium carbonate, or pearl ash, is somewhat alkaline, so additional neutralizers are necessary when you are formulating with it: 20 parts of pearl ash require 17 parts of boric acid for neutralization, or 85 percent. So to neutralize 2.5 ounces of carbonate, you'll need 2.1 ounces (60 grams) of boric acid. Dissolve the powdered boric acid in 4 ounces of hot water, and add after the paste has been diluted with water. Remember, you'll still need to add the standard 20 percent boric or citric acid solution (to neutralize the excess potassium hydroxide) as well.

This difficulty can be overcome in two ways. A few ounces of ethanol or isopropyl alcohol added to the water help liquefy the paste. Or make a less concentrated solution by adding more water. After the paste dissolves, boil the solution until the extra water evaporates; this will require a "before and after" weighing of the soap pot to determine the soap's concentration.

If you're not in a hurry, the paste will dissolve if it is left alone in gently simmering water, covered with a lid. Depending on the formulation, this may take an hour or more, but it's easy, and no foam is produced in the process.

Depending on how concentrated you wish to make the soap solution, you may need to transfer the paste to a larger pot for dilution. For example, 5 pounds of paste diluted with 10 pounds of water yields a liquid soap with a viscosity typical of the soap found in rest-room dispensers. That's a total of 15 pounds, or approximately 2 gallons. Use the 5-gallon double-boiler pot for these larger quantities. The soap is now neutral, so the lye won't affect the pot if it isn't stainless steel or enamel. Just make certain the pot isn't rusty.

9 Neutralize the Soap

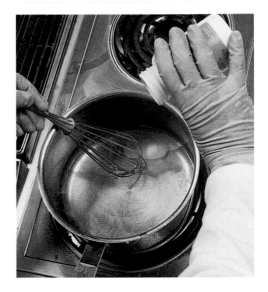

After the soap has been cooked and diluted, you'll need to add "buffers" to bring the pH down to neutral; neutral soap has a pH of 9.5 to 10. This is necessary because every recipe in this book has

Foaming is sometimes a nuisance when the soap is whisked into the hot water. A simple antidote for unwanted foam? Fill a spray bottle with isopropyl alcohol: A few short spritzes will subdue even the most menacing heads of froth. Take care to keep this spray away from open flames.

been formulated with a slight excess of potassium hydroxide to ensure that all free fatty acids are neutralized. As an interesting aside, the water used to dilute the paste actually lowers the pH; when 4 ounces of pH 10.35 paste are diluted with 6 ounces of water, the pH drops to 10.

But more than water is needed to neutralize soap. The neutralizers readily available for home soapmakers are citric acid, boric acid, and borax. These buffers should never be added directly to soap in their powdered form because localized concentrations of citric or boric acid, in particular, can throw soap out of solution and create a "snow flurry" of white flakes suspended in the clear soap. (These "snow flurries" will disappear if the soap is brought to a boil and stirred.)

➲ Dissolve neutralizers in water before adding them to liquid soap. To create a 20 percent buffer solution, add 2 ounces of citric or boric acid to 8 ounces of boiling distilled water. Stir until dissolved. Boric acid will precipitate out of solution when it is allowed to cool, so reheat it before adding to the soap solution.

➲ More borax is needed to neutralize a given amount of soap, compared with citric and boric acid, so a more concentrated buffer solution will be needed. Create this 33 percent solution by adding 3 ounces of borax to 6 ounces of boiling distilled water. If you intend to use borax as a thickener, forgo the addition of any neutralizers.

You'll find specifics on how much neutralizer to use per pound of soap on page 42.

10 Add Dyes and Fragrances

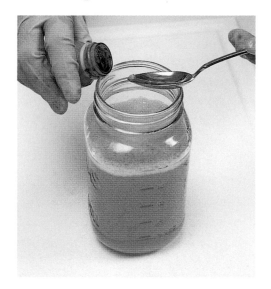

The ideal time for adding dye and fragrance to the soap is immediately after dilution and neutralization, while the soap is still near the boiling point. Fragrances won't disperse in cold soap; they'll just float as a greasy layer on the soap's surface.

Fragrances (whether essential oils or synthetics) can be added all at once into the hot liquid, then stirred thoroughly to aid their dispersal. Dyes should be added a little at a time, because a little color goes a long way in a clear liquid.

After the soap solution has cooled, you'll notice that the essential oils or fragrance oils have caused some clouding in the soap. This is because these oils aren't completely soluble even when stirred thoroughly into the hottest of soap bases. Essential oils cause more clouding than fragrance oils because fragrance oils have been purposefully formulated with solvents that help minimize clouding. The good news is that clouding will usually dissipate within a few days if the solution is allowed to settle.

Use only water-soluble or glycerin-based dyes for liquid soap. Oil-based dyes will cloud the finished soap. Water-based dyes will disperse evenly in hot or cold soap.

If you wish to add preservatives, the best time is while the soap solution is still hot; this allows for a homogenous dispersal of the preservative. Specifics on preservative amounts are given on page 43.

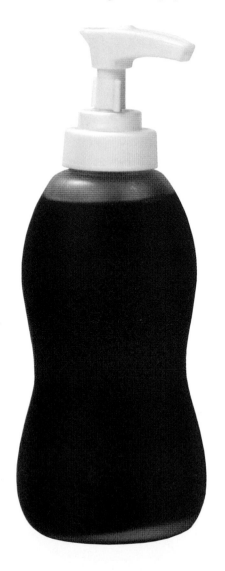

11 Sequester

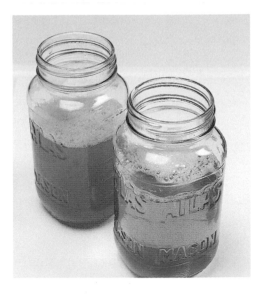

Pour the cooled soap into bottles, screw on lids, and allow the soap to stand for a week or two. This resting phase is called sequestering, a word that comes from the Latin word *sequestrare,* meaning "to remove, lay aside, or separate." Clouding caused by the addition of fragrances into the liquid should disappear during this time.

In addition, sequestering will clear up the minor clouding caused by insoluble fatty acid soaps. (This minor clouding may be barely noticeable, but the soap will appear "brighter" after a week of sequestering.) Even though liquid soaps are formulated without oils high in stearic and palmitic acids (the fatty acids responsible for forming insoluble soaps), all oils contain some percentage of both. Olive oil, for example, contains 7 percent

◄ Be sure to sequester the soap for at least a week to allow cloudiness to dissipate.

palmitic and 2 percent stearic acid. Coconut oil is made up of 9 percent palmitic and 2 percent stearic acid. These small percentages are enough to cause slight cloudiness. During the sequestering phase, the insoluble particles coalesce and precipitate to the bottom of the container; they will appear as a thin milky layer. The clear liquid can then be decanted or siphoned off.

The best place to sequester soap is a cool location, such as a basement. Clear glass or clear plastic containers work best for sequestering because the progress of the soap can be monitored. Commercial soapmakers actually age the soap for several days in a refrigerated room; it's then run through a filter that traps the precipitated insoluble substances. Obviously, the home soapmaker won't have access to a filtration system, but sequestering makes a marked difference in the brightness and clarity of the soap. *Note:* If you use borax as an emulsifier or thickener, add it to the liquid soap *after* sequestering. Otherwise, the insoluble soaps won't precipitate out of the more concentrated soap solution.

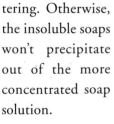

USING SEQUESTERING AGENTS

If your soap remains cloudy after 2 weeks of sequestering, you probably mismeasured the initial amounts of oil and lye or failed to thoroughly cook the paste. Not much can be done to correct cloudy soap once it's been diluted, but you might try adding some sequestering agents to help clarify the stock.

Sequestering agents lower the cloud point of a solution — that is, the point at which insolubles coalesce and cause milkiness. Sequestering agents available to home soapmakers are alcohol, glycerin, and sugar solutions. A few ounces of any of these solvents can correct minor clouding; however, excess solvent can dampen the lathering ability of the soap. More details on sequestering agents are given on page 45.

the alcohol/lye method

Commercial potassium soaps are stirred continuously and cooked at high temperatures to completely neutralize all fatty acids. It's impossible to duplicate these conditions at home using the paste method, largely because of the difficulty of stirring the taffylike soap. But by dissolving the soap in alcohol, home soapmakers can come much closer to producing commercial-quality potassium soap.

Modified from a technique first introduced in my book *Making Transparent Soap,* the alcohol/lye method has several advantages over the paste method: It's easier (no stirring), faster (2 hours versus 3 hours cooking time), and yields a somewhat clearer finished soap. If you don't want alcohol in your finished soap, it can be evaporated out of solution.

Alcohols are solvents. When ethanol or isopropyl alcohol is added to an oil and lye mix, the alcohol accelerates saponification by lowering the surface tension between the oil and the caustic solution. When added in large enough quantities, alcohol dissolves soap completely; what remains is a clear amber broth. As this broth cooks at a gentle boil, the mechanical action of the boiling substitutes for stirring.

Either ethanol or isopropyl alcohol can be used for the alcohol/lye method. Ethanol is an excellent solvent and is odorless as well. However, it can be expensive unless purchased in gallon containers through scientific supply houses. By comparison, isopropyl alcohol is inexpensive and readily available; the downside is its strong, characteristic odor. Ideally, the isopropyl alcohol should be at strengths of 90 percent or over; weaker concentrations introduce too much water, which consequently slows the saponification rate. Whichever alcohol you choose, always have a little more on hand than what the recipe calls for. This reserve will be used to replace any alcohol lost through evaporation.

A note for crafters of transparent soap bars: The no-stir alcohol method works for these soaps, as well.

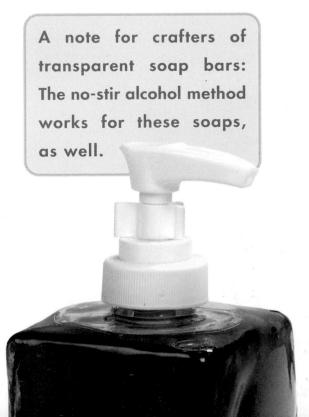

1 Make a Cap and Prepare the Double Boiler

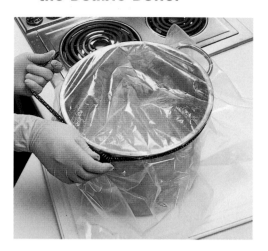

Before measuring the oils and lye solution, prepare a plastic "cap" for your soap pot from plastic sheeting. Cut the plastic into two pieces large enough to allow for 5 to 6 inches of additional drape beyond the circumference of the pot. After the alcohol is added to the soap stock, the plastic will be tightly secured to the rim of the pot with bungee cords.

➲ Fill the 5-gallon canning pot with 3 to 4 inches of water and bring to a slow boil on the back burner. This pot functions as the bottom of a double boiler.

2 Heat the Fats and Oils

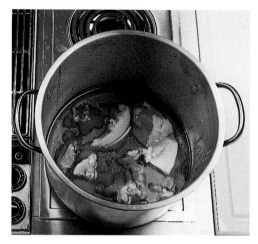

Weigh the fats and oils, then add them to the soap pot, and melt over medium heat. Continue heating until the temperature reaches 160°F (71°C).

SAFETY PRECAUTIONS FOR USING ALCOHOL

Alcohol is flammable. Commonsense precautions must be taken when this solvent is used. The alcohol/lye method is not recommended for soapmakers working over a gas range.

➪ Keep all alcohol away from open flames. Electric ranges don't pose the same hazards as gas ranges. If you only have a gas range, you might instead try cooking the soap on a hot plate. Be sure the hot plate's electrical cord is in working condition, and plug it directly into an outlet; do not use an extension cord.

➪ Make sure the work space has adequate ventilation.

➪ Equip your area with a working fire extinguisher. You may also wish to keep on hand a spray bottle filled with water. Alcohol is soluble in water, so a spray aimed at the base of any flames will quench the fire by diluting the alcohol.

3 Add the Lye-Water Solution

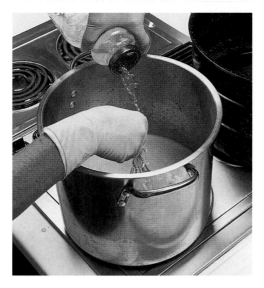

4 Mix in the Alcohol

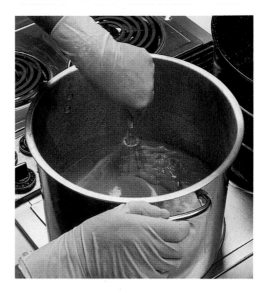

Weigh the potassium hydroxide and distilled water. In an alkali-resistant container, add the hydroxide to the water and stir until dissolved. **Then pour this hot solution directly into the 160°F (71°C) oils and stir for a minute or two.**

Add the alcohol directly to the oil and lye mix. Initially, the solution separates into two layers — you'll notice the oily layer swirling on top. Stir for a few minutes until the solution appears homogenous. Stop stirring, and check for the reappearance of the oily layer. If it appears, continue stirring until the solution is uniform.

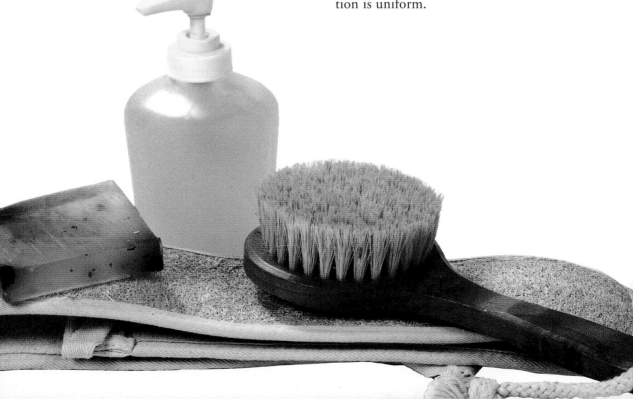

5 Cover the Pot

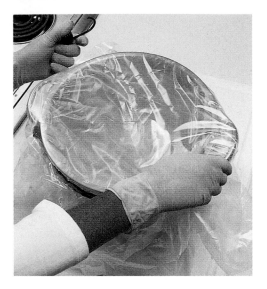

When the mixture has become homogenous, cover the soap pot with one of the plastic sheets. Secure it to the rim of the soap pot with a tightly stretched bungee cord — the tighter the fit, the less evaporation. Be careful not to pierce the plastic with the bungee hooks.

➲ Reduce any slack in the plastic by gently pulling the excess underneath the bungee cord; the soap pot should resemble a tight drumhead with ruffles around the sides.

➲ Repeat this procedure with the second sheet of plastic and the second bungee cord.

6 Weigh the Pot

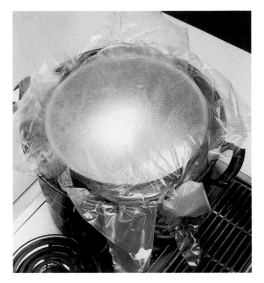

Before cooking the broth, weigh the soap pot. Include the weight of the plastic and bungee cords in this figure, which will be your baseline weight. **Over the course of the 2-hour cooking time, you'll occasionally remove the pot from the stove and weigh it to monitor how much alcohol is being lost to evaporation.**

> Always put on your protective goggles and gloves before handling any caustic substances or cooking soap paste.

7 Cook the Paste

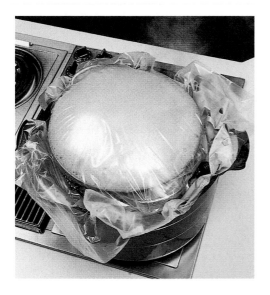

Through the plastic, watch for the boiling of the paste; this should happen within a few minutes. Then adjust the heat so that the solution maintains a gentle, steady boil for the next 2 hours. The emphasis is on a gentle boil; vigorous boiling serves only to hasten the evaporation of alcohol.

The expanding steam and alcohol will stretch the plastic, causing it to balloon above the rim of the pot. This may look a bit scary, but the plastic won't rupture because of its thickness. This mushrooming will cause the excess plastic "frill" around the pot to be pulled under the bungee cords. Make sure it doesn't pull completely out from under the cords, allowing alcohol to escape. If necessary, tighten the plastic by pulling it back under the bungee cords.

8 Weigh the Pot

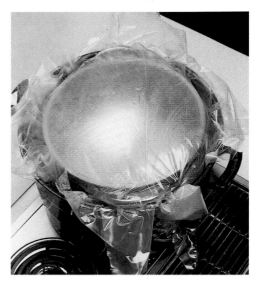

In 20 or 30 minutes, remove the pot from the double boiler and weigh the soap pot. Determine the alcohol loss by subtracting the new weight from the original baseline weight. Please note that as long as the solution remains fluid, it isn't necessary to add alcohol, even if a few ounces have evaporated. When the solution develops a frothy head of foam, however, the solution is beginning to revert to a paste. Now is the time to add more alcohol. If the baseline weight and the new weight vary by 8 ounces, for example, unwrap the plastic and add 8 more ounces of alcohol. If the solution has lost 14 ounces, add 14 more ounces of alcohol.

➲ Reweigh the pot every half hour throughout the 2-hour cooking time. If the plastic is tight and the solution isn't cooking at a high boil, you might not need to replace any alcohol whatsoever.

9 Test for Excess Fatty Acids

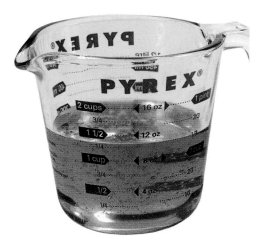

Your soap should be neutral after 2 hours of continuous cooking. Test for the presence of excess fatty acids in an alcohol-based soap using the same method you'd use to test a paste: **Dilute a few ounces of soap in a few ounces of water, and allow the solution to cool.** If the solution shows more than slight cloudiness, continue cooking. If dense cloudiness persists after 3 hours of cooking, consult chapter 8.

CREATING AN ALCOHOL-FREE SOAP PASTE

Alcohol can be left in the finished soap if you so desire. It enhances the clarity and brightness of the finished soap. Essential oils are less likely to cloud soap containing alcohol, because alcohol acts as a solvent.

If you wish to remove the alcohol, do so after the soap sample has tested clear in cooled water. Remove the plastic from the top of the pot, but leave the pot inside the double boiler. Bring the water in the bottom pot to a fast boil. As the alcohol in the soap solution evaporates, the soap thickens and foams. Continue cooking until the solution becomes a paste; this can then be diluted with water following the procedure outlined in the paste method.

10 Dilute the Soap Broth

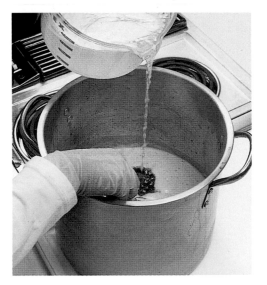

11 Neutralize the Soap

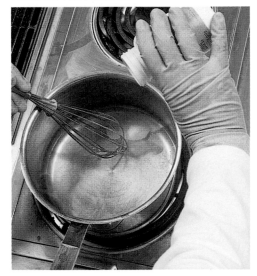

Bring water to a boil, then add the soap paste. (See chart on page 42 for dilution guidelines.) Another advantage of the alcohol-lye method over the paste method is that the broth dissolves instantly in hot water — no breaking up of paste chunks will be necessary. Keep in mind that a little less water will be needed for dilution to compensate for the alcohol in solution. For example, if the recipe requires 1 pound of alcohol, use 1 pound less water when diluting the soap.

If allowed to cool, the broth hardens into a clear paste. This can be wrapped up and refrigerated for later use. Alcohol-based paste dissolves quite rapidly when added to boiling water because of the solvency of the alcohol.

▶ Always use distilled or soft water in your soap recipes for best results.

Neutralize the solution by adding borax, citric acid, or boric acid solution. To create a 20 percent buffer solution, add 2 ounces of citric or boric acid to 8 ounces of boiling distilled water. Stir until dissolved. Boric acid will precipitate out of solution when allowed to cool, so reheat before adding to the soap solution. If you prefer to use borax, see the information on page 30 for the paste method.

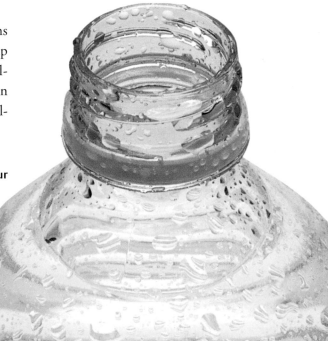

12 Add Dyes and Fragrances

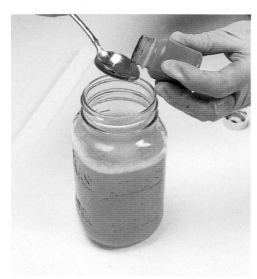

13 Sequester

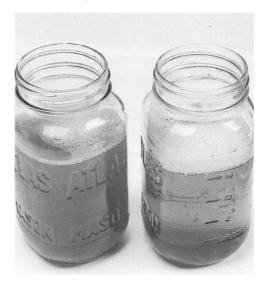

Add the dyes and fragrances to the hot soap stock. Remember: Do not use oil-based dyes, which can cloud the soap. Preservatives should also be added now while the soap is still hot (see page 43 for preservatives). Whisk thoroughly for optimum dispersal.

Sequester alcohol-based soaps in covered jars in the same manner as soaps made with the paste method: Allow the diluted liquid to settle for 1 to 2 weeks until the insoluble soaps and the cloudiness caused by fragrance oils settle out of the solution.

Whether you followed the paste method or the alcohol/lye method, after the soap has been sequestered, it's ready to use!

guidelines for dilution

The previous sections were intended as a broad overview of the two basic liquid soapmaking methods. You're certain to be nagged by many unanswered questions. Exactly how much boric acid is necessary to neutralize soap? How many ounces of sulfonated castor oil are needed for superfatting? Just what is a 20 percent soap solution?

The following information will answer your questions. These guidelines apply to all soap formulations in this book

Dilution Rates

In commercial liquid soapmaking, soap concentrations are referred to as percentages of "true" or "actual" soap. Actual soap means the combined weight of the oils and dry hydroxide. Water and any other additives in the formulation aren't counted. Water accounts for approximately 35 to 40 percent of the weight in a potassium soap formulation; the remaining 60 to 65 percent of the paste is "actual" soap.

The recipes in this book all yield approximately 6 pounds of paste. If, for example, you dilute all 6 pounds down to a 20 percent soap concentration, you'll see from the chart on page 42 that a 20 percent solution requires 2 pounds of water per 1 pound of paste. Likewise, 6 pounds of paste requires 12 pounds of water, for a grand total of 18 pounds of finished soap.

The dilution rates range from 15 to 40 percent for a reason: At concentrations much below 15 percent, the soap becomes too thin to lather effectively, and at progressively higher concentrations, the solution begins coagulating back into paste. Because of the soluble nature of coconut oil, 100 percent coconut oil soaps can form the most highly concentrated solutions at 40 percent actual soap to 60 percent water. Soft oils form soaps that congeal at lower concentrations, starting at about 20 to 25 percent actual soap. Blends of coconut oil and soft oils will therefore yield soaps that require dilutions of approximately 25 to 35 percent actual soap.

If you follow the alcohol/lye method and choose to leave the alcohol in solution, always discount the weight of the alcohol from the weight of water needed for dilution; otherwise, the finished soap will be thinner than planned. All recipes require 20 ounces of alcohol, so subtract 20 ounces from the total water weight, unless a few ounces of alcohol have evaporated during the 2-hour cooking time.

Some fine-tuning may be necessary to create a proper concentration. A solution is too concentrated if a sticky, viscous layer develops on the surface of the finished soap. The thicker the layer, the more water is needed for dilution. However, stronger soap concentrations without the layering problem can be created by the use of borax. The addition of 2 tablespoons of a 33 percent borax solution per pound of diluted soap emulsifies the soap and helps prevent the formation of layers. Read more about the use of borax for emulsifying and thickening on the facing page.

A Guide to Dilution Percentages

Percent Actual Soap	Water Added per Pound of Paste
15 percent	48 ounces (3 lb)
20 percent	32 ounces (2 lb)
25 percent	22 ounces (1 lb 6 oz)
30 percent	16 ounces (1 lb)
35 percent	12 ounces
40 percent	9 ounces

using additives

One of the beauties of liquid soapmaking is that a single soap base can be modified with different additives to create completely different finished soaps. Here are some ideas and general guidelines; note that, with the exception of neutralizers, all additives are strictly optional.

Neutralizers

One pound of soap paste requires approximately ¾ ounce (or 1½ tablespoons) of a 20 percent boric or citric acid solution, or ¾ ounce of a 33 percent borax solution, for neutralization. (See page 30 for instructions on making acid solutions.) All the formulations in this book yield about 6 pounds of paste, so approximately 4½ ounces (or 9 tablespoons) of either borax or acid (citric, boric) solution is necessary.

Borax is a mild alkali (pH 9.2), not an acid. Its effectiveness as a buffer is due to the fact that its pH is lower than the pH of soap (9.5–10). Because it isn't an acid, borax won't throw soap out of solution, and it can consequently be added to either hot or cold liquid soap. Remember, too, that no neutralizers will be necessary when you use borax as a thickener.

The amounts of neutralizers for the recipes in this book are approximate amounts only. Differences in types of oils, cooking time, dilution rates, and other variables all affect the pH of the finished soap. The best way to fine-tune this process is to use phenolphthalein. Instructions are given on page 14.

Preservatives

Thoroughly neutralized soaps with fresh, clean-smelling oils should need no preservatives. If you feel more comfortable adding preservatives, use a scant teaspoon of rosemary extract or mixed-tocopherol vitamin E per pound of soap paste. Stir into hot, diluted soap stock for optimal dispersal.

Superfatting

Sulfonated castor oil is the only superfatting agent suitable for liquid soap. Sulfonated castor oil lubricates like an oil but is completely water soluble; all other oils will cloud the soap because of the liberation of free fatty acids.

For every pound of dilute soap stock, superfat with approximately 1 percent sulfonated castor oil. For 12 pounds of liquid soap, for example, convert 12 pounds into ounces (12 x 16), then multiply by .01; 192 ounces soap will require 1.92 ounces, or approximately 4 tablespoons, of sulfonated castor oil.

Thickeners

As consumers, we're accustomed to thick, full-bodied liquid soaps. This thickness isn't inherent in the soap itself but is created by surfactants, cellulose derivatives, carrageenan, and other additives. Commercial soaps are commonly 20 percent soap and 80 percent water. At that concentration, soap is quite watery if formulated without viscosity builders. Even though thin soap cleans as well as thick, many of us still prefer fuller-bodied soaps.

Borax. One way to enhance soap viscosity is to add borax.

Borax is the "silver bullet" of liquid soapmaking. It enhances and stabilizes foam, softens hard water, buffers pH, and acts as a preservative. Borax is also invaluable for creating more concentrated soap solutions because of its ability to both emulsify and thicken.

Different soap bases begin congealing at different concentrations. This congealing is first apparent as a gooey "crust" on the surface of the soap solution. In time, this thickening extends further down into the body of the soap until the entire containerful has coagulated. Olive oil and other soft oils congeal in concentrations as low as 20 to 25 percent actual soap to water; coconut oil begins layering at much higher saturations — approximately 40 percent soap to 60 percent water. The home soapmaker can overcome these limitations by adding 2 to 3 tablespoons of a 33 percent borax solution per pound of dilute soap. The borax actually emulsifies the solution, creating a homogenous solution free of a thick upper "crust." You are now free to experiment with different concentrations of soap than the soap might otherwise allow.

Borax is also a viscosity modifier, or thickening agent. Chemically, sodium borate cross-links with hydroxide molecules to form thicker soap. Interestingly, this tendency is very marked when borax is added to a soap high in soft oils, which makes borax an ideal additive for gel soapmaking (see chapter 5). Little or no thickening, however, can be observed when borax is added to a soap formulation high in coconut oil, which is highly soluble. Borax will emulsify coconut oil soaps but not thicken them.

One other limitation to the effectiveness of borax as a thickener is that it works best in soaps of higher concentration. The thinner and less concentrated the soap solution, the smaller the effect borax has on viscosity.

For thickening soap solutions high in soft oils, create a 33 percent borax solution by dissolving 4 ounces of borax in 8 ounces of boiling water. Add to diluted soap stock at a rate of ½ to 1 ounce of solution per 1 pound of soap stock. Start with ½ ounce and test the viscosity. If you desire a thicker soap, add another ½ ounce. The more borax, the thicker the emulsion. But past a certain point, the soap progressively clouds with increasing additions of borax; this is due to both a lower pH and an elevated cloud point and is particularly evident in fragranced soap. When borax is used as a thickening agent, it's best to add it to cold soap because changes in viscosity are more apparent in cold solutions than in hot.

When using borax as an emulsifier or thickener, add it after the soap has been sequestered — unless you're satisfied with the clarity of the newly diluted soap. Insoluble soaps won't be able to settle out of the more concentrated solutions created by the addition of borax. If your sequestered soap has formed a crust, remove it and remelt the soap in a microwave or double boiler. Stir this solution into the clear sequestered liquid, and then add borax.

MAKING CONCENTRATED SOAP SOLUTIONS

True potassium soaps lack the thickness of commercial soaps. Many first-time makers of potassium soaps are surprised at how thin a potassium soap solution can seem.

Homemade potassium soaps that can't be thickened with borax can be thickened by modifying the cooking method for gels outlined in chapter 5. For every pound of paste, add 2 ounces of alcohol and 4 ounces of glycerin. Cook the paste, glycerin, and alcohol over medium heat until the paste dissolves; another ounce or two of alcohol may be needed to compensate for evaporation. Now stir in 6 ounces of water. Test the viscosity of the liquid by spooning a small sample into a bowl and covering it with regular plastic wrap to prevent evaporation.

When the solution cools, you'll have a "snapshot" of your entire batch. If the solution's too thick, add a couple of ounces of water and test again. If it's too thin, continue boiling the solution, testing every few minutes until you're satisfied with the finished soap.

Calgon can be used in much the same manner as borax. The only drawback is that its color and fragrance become your soap's color and fragrance.

Gums and seaweed extracts. Other natural additives for thickening soap include carrageenan and cellulose derivatives. Many of these natural extracts perform best in lower pH solutions and don't work as well in high-pH true soaps. They often contain substances that cause minor clouding in the body of the liquid soap; one exception is purified xanthan gum. If you wish to experiment with carrageenan or other gums, add the gum at a rate of 1 percent of the total weight of the diluted soap. These thickeners clump when added directly to a liquid, so make a "slurry" by mixing the gum in a few ounces of glycerin before adding it to the soap.

Sequestering Agents

Soap suffering from minor cloudiness caused by excess fatty acids or essential oils can often be cured with alcohol, glycerin, and sugar solutions added to diluted soap at a rate of roughly 5 percent. For example, 10 pounds of slightly milky soap, or 160 ounces, can be mixed with up to 8 ounces of a sequestrant (160 x .05 = 8). Five percent is a somewhat arbitrary number; start with less, then add more if needed. Sequestrants in excess of 5 percent can be used, but remember that too much will dampen the soap's foaming action.

Alcohol, glycerin, and sugar solution can be added alone or in combination. You might try a 1:1:1 blend of all three. An effective sugar solution can be concocted by boiling 1 pound of water, then adding 1½ pounds of sugar; bring the solution back to a boil, and cook it until all the sugar has dissolved.

Reheat the soap solution before adding sequestrants. When mixed with cold soap, the sequestrants take a day or so before a change in clarity becomes noticeable. You'll see the effects immediately when you add a sequestrant to hot soap. Nonetheless, it's a good idea to give the soap a few more days of sequestering time, because it will continue to clarify after solvents have been incorporated.

Note: Besides its usefulness as a sequestering agent, glycerin is an excellent moisturizer, humectant, and lather booster. Add 1 to 2 ounces of glycerin to every pound of diluted liquid soap for extra emollience and mildness.

Herbs

If you love herbs, as many soapmakers do, one of your first liquid soap experiments will probably involve the dilution of soap paste with herb-infused water. Because lavender is an excellent hair conditioner, isn't lavender water the logical choice for a shampoo base? Yes, if it's added to a low-pH detergent shampoo. But the higher pH of true soap doesn't react kindly with herbal infusions; the infusions tend to turn brown and cloudy. Instead, use herbal essential oils. Shampoo formulations, in particular, benefit from these oils.

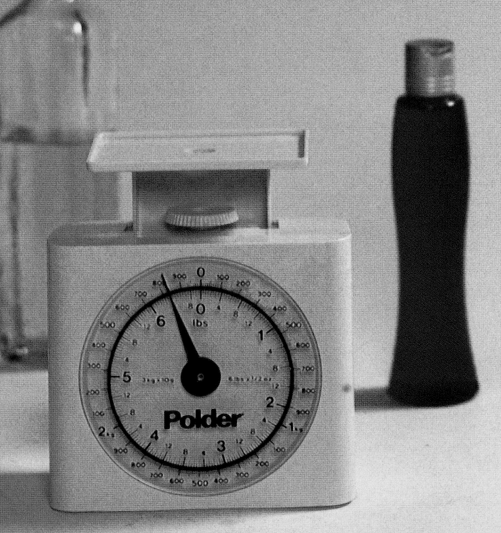

formulating
(3) blends

Add goat grease to a liberal amount of spruce ash and mix well. This is one of the first recorded "recipes" for potassium soap, written some two thousand years ago in the *Historiae Naturalis* by Pliny the Elder of Rome. The salve of goat grease and spruce ash was used by the Teutons not for washing but for smoothing and "styling" hair, as well as for dyeing. It wasn't until A.D. 200 that the Romans discovered the cleansing properties of soap.

These days, there are many different types of soap on the market. But why use a synthetic detergent when you can create all-natural versions in your own kitchen? This chapter will get you started with some basic recipes and provide information for formulating liquid soap from scratch.

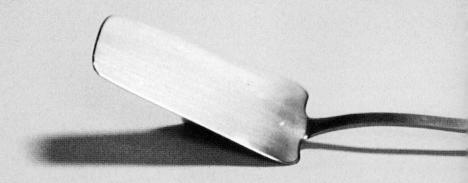

the first liquid soaps

Early soapmakers learned to make sodium soaps by adding common salt to a potassium soap base. Because of their ease of storage and transport, sodium soaps were the only soaps available until the 1930s, when liquid soaps first appeared.

These early liquids, however, were formulated for industrial and institutional markets. Not until the late 1970s was the Softsoap brand introduced: the first liquid soap for personal, in-home use. Packaged in an attractive pump dispenser, Softsoap's overnight success triggered a mad scramble for market share by every major soap producer in the country.

Softsoap and most liquid soaps on the market today are synthetic detergents; the notable exception is Dr. Bronner's brand liquid soap. From a mass-production standpoint, synthetic soaps have much to recommend them: longer shelf lives, more consistency in the raw materials, and more stability when exposed to extremes of temperature.

▶ Proper oil measurements will ensure soap that is rich and has good lather.

Simple and Natural

The vast majority of home soapmakers today prefer more traditional soapmaking methods that rely on simple, pure ingredients and a minimum of synthetic additives. "Old-fashioned" potassium soaps are a perfect fit: They're formulated with inexpensive vegetable oils, require little or nothing in the way of preservatives, and allow much room for experimentation and improvisation.

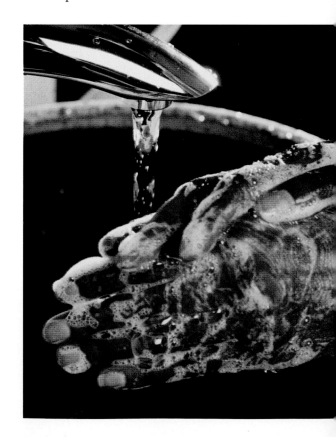

formulating your own soap

Soapmaking is an art as well as a science. The calculation of lye solutions, measurement of ingredients and temperatures, proper cooking, and cure times are all science. The blending of oils and additives as well as dyeing and fragrancing are all art.

Oil Blends

The most important art in liquid soap-making lies in proper oil blending. Potassium soaps are somewhat easier than sodium bar soaps in this respect because liquids are formulated almost exclusively with coconut oil and soft oils. Coconut oil forms the backbone of all liquid soaps, typically accounting for 70 to 90 percent of a formulation. It produces a high, foamy lather and performs well in salt and hard waters, but a 100 percent coconut oil soap is drying to the skin. This is why coconut oil is usually "toned down" with at least 10 percent of a soft oil, which lends mildness and emollience. On the other hand, a 100 percent soft oil liquid soap produces a stingy, low-lather soap and needs to be fortified with a minimum of 10 percent coconut oil.

Many soft oils are available to the soapmaker. For a discussion of different soft oils for soapmaking, see chapter 1. Please consult the Soapmaking Properties of Common Fats and Oils chart on page 6 to find out which oil will best fit your purpose.

Where crystal-clear soaps are desired, hard fats such as palm oil and tallow should be used sparingly if at all. The palmitic and stearic acids in these oils form insoluble soaps that have a "milky" appearance. The chart on page 5 will help you select oils low in these two acids. Lanolin and jojoba also cause cloudiness not because they form insoluble soaps but because they are technically waxes and contain a high percentage of substances that do not saponify. When formulating with cloud-causing oils or waxes, begin with small amounts — approximately 3 to 5 percent of the oil total. If crystal clarity is not important to you, larger quantities of these oils and waxes can be used in your formulas.

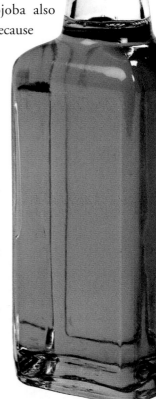

NO-FUSS BLENDING TECHNIQUE

Here's an easy, timesaving technique for developing soap blends. If you wish to create a soap combining coconut oil, castor oil, and jojoba, for example, weigh out a pound of each oil, then mix up three separate lye solutions. Mix each oil with its corresponding lye solution and stir until thickened. Spoon into three 1-quart mason jars and place the jars in a double boiler. Cook the three pastes until they are neutral, then dilute them separately, using the same proportion of water for each. Finding that perfect blend is now a simple matter of mixing the three soaps in various combinations and testing until you're satisfied. Be sure to keep notes!

Alkali Needed to Saponify Common Oils/Fats/Waxes

Oil, Fat, or Wax	% of Sodium Hydroxide (NaOH)	% of Potassium Hydroxide (KOH)	Oil, Fat, or Wax	% of Sodium Hydroxide (NaOH)	% of Potassium Hydroxide (KOH)
Sweet almond oil	13.7	19.2	Olive	13.6	19
			Palm	14.2	19.9
Avocado oil	13.4	18.7	Palm kernel	15.7	22
Babassu oil	17.6	24.6			
Canola oil	13.7	19.2	Peanut	13.7	19.2
Castor oil	12.8	17.9	Rosin	13	18.2
Cocoa butter	13.8	19.3	Safflower	13.7	19.2
			Sesame	13.4	18.7
Coconut oil	19	26.6	Shea butter	12	18
Corn oil	13.7	19.2			
Hemp oil	13.7	19.2	Soybean	13.6	19
Jojoba oil	7	9.8	Tallow	14.1	19.6
Lard	13.9	19.5	Wheat germ	13.2	18.5
Lanolin	7.6	10.6			

Calculating Lye Proportions

Each soapmaking oil requires a different amount of sodium or potassium hydroxide for neutralization; this amount is the saponification value. Saponification values are numbers that are converted mathematically into percentages of hydroxide per pound of oil. With simplicity in mind, the percentages alone are listed in the chart on the facing page. For each oil needed, convert the pounds of oil into ounces, then multiply by the percentage of potassium hydroxide needed for neutralization. Add all the numbers together for the total amount of potassium hydroxide needed for the recipe.

Let's say you want an oil blend consisting of 2 pounds of coconut oil, 1 pound of canola oil, and .5 pound of castor oil.

For coconut oil:
32 x .266 = 8.5 ounces KOH
For canola oil:
16 x .192 = 3.07 ounces KOH
For castor oil:
8 x .179 = 1.43 ounces KOH
Add all three hydroxide numbers together (8.5 + 3.07 + 1.43) for a total of 13 ounces of potassium hydroxide.

You'll overalkalize, however, to ensure that all free fatty acids are neutralized. The recipes in this book are calculated in excess of approximately 10 percent potassium hydroxide. Multiply 13 x .1, and the hydroxide total equals 1.3 ounces.

Potassium hydroxide solutions typically contain 50 percent more water than sodium hydroxide solutions. For every pound of dry potassium hydroxide, multiply by 3; for example, 14.1 ounces potassium hydroxide requires 42 ounces of water.

Your finished formula for 2 pounds of coconut oil, 1 pound of canola oil, and .5 pound of castor oil is now:

• 32 ounces coconut oil
• 16 ounces canola oil
• 8 ounces castor oil
• 14.3 ounces potassium hydroxide
• 42 ounces soft or distilled water

To neutralize, just remember that each pound of finished paste (at 10 percent excess alkali) requires approximately 1½ tablespoons of a 20 percent boric or citric acid solution, or 1½ tablespoons of a 33 percent borax solution. These amounts are only approximations; the use of phenolphthalein (see page 14 for instructions) is the only method for guaranteeing truly neutral soap.

basic soap recipes

Using the instructions in chapter 2 as your guide, you can use the following formulas for basic hand and body soaps. These are "no-frills" recipes; if you wish to enhance your soap with moisturizers, foam boosters, or other additives, refer to the Additives Guide on page 60 for ideas, or let your imagination guide you!

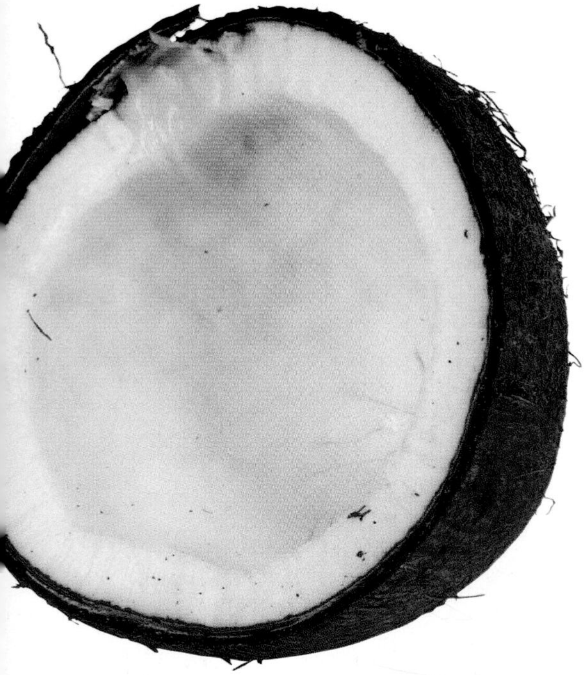

You'll need soft oil — such as olive, almond, canola, safflower, or soy — for most of these recipes. Two rules apply to all of the recipes in this chapter:

If using the alcohol/lye method to make your soap, add 20 ounces ethanol or isopropyl alcohol to the oils and lye solution.

To neutralize the soap, add 4½ ounces of a 20 percent boric or citric acid solution, or 4½ ounces of a 33 percent borax solution. *Note:* If you use borax as an emulsifer or thickener, no neutralizers will be necessary.

100% Coconut Oil Soap

This soap is high-foaming and excellent for use in hard and salt waters. Not recommended for dry skin.

Oil
48 ounces coconut oil

Lye solution
14 ounces potassium hydroxide
42 ounces soft or distilled water

Mild Coconut Oil Soap

Another high-foaming formula, this soap is milder because it contains soft oils.

Oils
35 ounces coconut oil
13 ounces soft oil of choice

Lye solution
13 ounces potassium hydroxide
39 ounces soft or distilled water

▲ Coconut oil is the basis of all liquid soaps, but you should blend it with a soft oil to prevent drying of your skin.

Creamy Coconut Oil Soap

A terrific medium-foaming soap, with rich lather.

Oils
> 23 ounces coconut oil
> 25 ounces soft oil of choice

Lye solution
> 12 ounces potassium hydroxide
> 36 ounces soft or distilled water

Supermild Soap

Very mild, emollient lather, though not as high-foaming as the soaps in the other recipes on these two pages.

Oils
> 10 ounces coconut oil
> 39 ounces soft oil of choice

Lye solution
> 11 ounces potassium hydroxide
> 33 ounces soft or distilled water

High-Foaming Rosin Soap

Beautiful amber liquid with abundant, moisturizing lather.

Oils
> 30 ounces coconut oil
> 9 ounces soft oil of choice
> 7 ounces rosin

Lye solution
> 12 ounces potassium hydroxide
> 36 ounces soft or distilled water

High-Foaming Cold Cream Soap

Castor oil makes this soap produce lots of lather with a cold-cream, moisturizing finish. Great for dry skin.

Oils
> 35 ounces coconut oil
> 11 ounces castor oil
> 3 ounces palm oil or tallow

Lye solution
> 13 ounces potassium hydroxide
> 39 ounces soft or distilled water

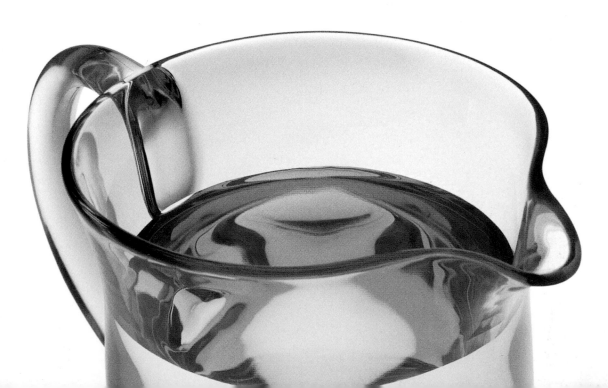

Liquid Soap with Palm Oil

Palm oil helps build "body" in liquid soap. Not quite as crystal clear as soft oil/coconut blend soaps, but great nonetheless.

Oils

- 18 ounces coconut oil
- 22 ounces soft oil of choice
- 5 ounces palm oil or tallow

Lye solution

- 11 ounces potassium hydroxide
- 33 ounces soft or distilled water

Castor Oil–Jojoba Moisturizing Soap

The high percentages of soft oil, castor oil, and jojoba make this soap exceptionally mild. The solventlike castor oil will also tone down the clouding effects of jojoba.

Oils

- 24 ounces coconut oil
- 10 ounces soft oil of choice
- 10 ounces castor oil
- 3 ounces jojoba

Lye solution

- 11 ounces potassium hydroxide
- 33 ounces soft or distilled water

Moisturizing Jojoba Soap

A very mild, moisturizing soap. Because jojoba contains some substances that do not saponify, this soap may not be quite as crystal clear as some other formulations.

Oils

- 16 ounces coconut oil
- 29 ounces soft oil of choice
- 3 ounces jojoba

Lye solution

- 11 ounces potassium hydroxide
- 33 ounces soft or distilled water

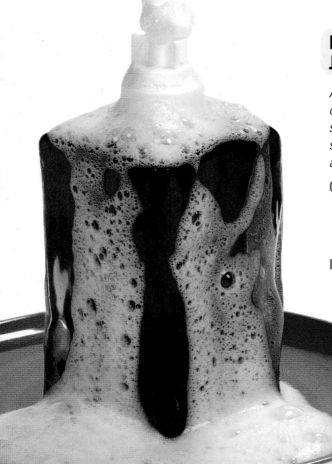

◄ **No matter which soft oil you choose, the soap will have cleansing properties that rival those of commercial soaps.**

Lanolin Soap

Lanolin, like jojoba, is chemically similar to our skin's own natural moisturizers. Lanolin contains many substances that do not saponify and tend to form a slight film on the surface of the finished soap. This film can be skimmed off or shaken back into solution.

Oils

16 ounces coconut oil
29 ounces soft oil of choice
3 ounces lanolin

Lye solution

11 ounces potassium hydroxide
33 ounces soft or distilled water

Castor Oil–Rosin Soap

The very first transparent soap bars were formulated with castor oil and rosin some two hundred years ago. These two ingredients impart exceptional clarity to liquid soap as well.

Oils

39 ounces coconut oil
6 ounces castor oil
4 ounces rosin

Lye solution

13 ounces potassium hydroxide
39 ounces soft or distilled water

▶ **If you have dry skin, try using lanolin or jojoba in your recipes.**

Remember to add the appropriate amount of ethanol or isopropyl alcohol if you're using the alcohol/lye method for any of these recipes. See page 41 for more information.

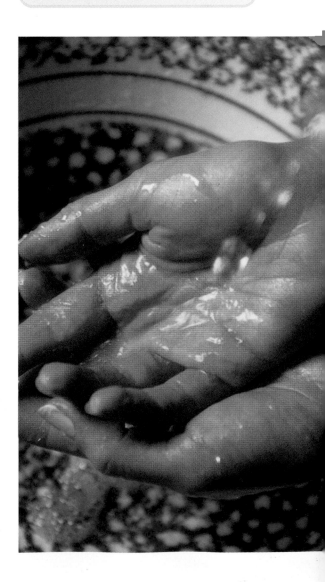

premium ④ natural shampoos

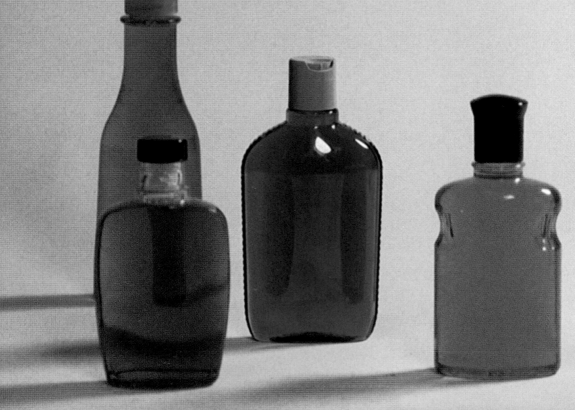

Liquid shampoo is a relative newcomer. Throughout history, if and when people washed their hair, they used bar soap. Liquid detergent shampoos were first introduced in 1930 and were followed by cream and liquid cream shampoos. A commercial "true soap" shampoo today will probably contain 25 percent coconut oil, a trace of olive oil, 15 percent alcohol, and 50 percent water and glycerol.

You can make a host of different shampoos simply by varying the types and proportions of oil. I've also included a section on additives that will improve the cleaning, conditioning, moisturizing, and shine-enhancing capabilities of your shampoos. As with other liquid soaps, you may also use dyes and fragrances to embellish your finished shampoos.

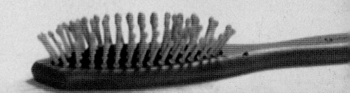

what does shampoo do?

To a certain extent, shampoos are glorified liquid soaps. The recipes in chapter 3 can be used as shampoos, and shampoo formulations can likewise substitute for liquid soap. Shampoos, however, do take a bit more care and thought to formulate, because creating a perfect shampoo involves the reconciliation of two opposing aims: cleansing and conditioning. An effective cleanser needs to *remove* deposits from the hair, whereas an effective conditioner needs to *deposit* additives on the hair.

Cleaning and Conditioning

Hair becomes "dirty" because of the buildup of sebum, the oily substance produced by the sebaceous glands contained in every hair follicle in the scalp. For shampoos to clean hair effectively, they must first penetrate the layer of sebum that coats the hair shaft. This is accomplished by using a preponderance of oils that contain short-chained fatty acid molecules; these small molecules dissolve the water-oil interface more rapidly than long-chained molecules, such as stearic acid. The most notable short-chained fatty acid is lauric acid, the predominant acid in coconut oil.

Conditioners are added to shampoos to counteract the damage done to hair by other hair preparations, especially bleach and dye. Conditioners fall into three classes: humectants, finishing agents, and emulsifiers. Humectants draw moisture from the air and hold it to the hair shaft. Humectants commonly used in commercial shampoos include glycerin, propylene glycol, sorbitol, and urea. Finishing agents such as balsam peru and isopropyl myristate leave a film on the hair, creating the "soft and shiny" look. Emulsifiers should be nonsticking and should disappear when rubbed between the hands. Emulsifiers homogenize the ingredients

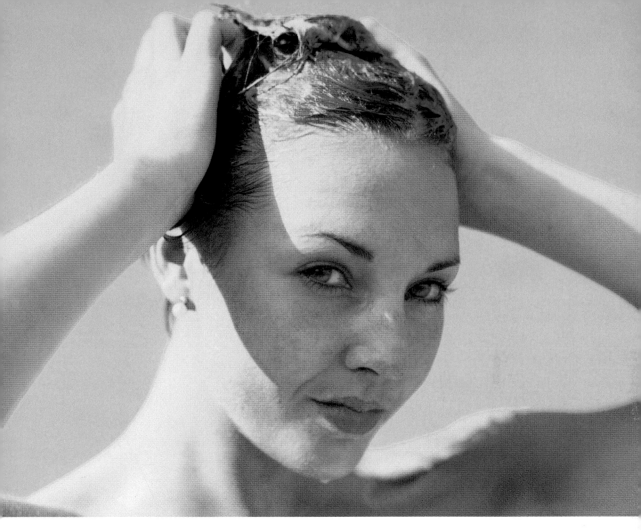

▲ While cleansing and conditioning might seem impossible to achieve with the same product, you can easily create shampoos that both clean your hair and improve its texture.

> The protein in human hair is very similar to wool protein, and early research on wool contributed greatly to our knowledge of the structure and properties of human hair.

in the soap and also boost the penetrating cleaning power of the soap by lowering surface tension. Alcohols, lanolin, spermaceti, glycerin, mineral oil, and perfumes are common emulsifiers.

The protein keratin constitutes about 80 percent of human hair. Many shampoos and conditioners on the market contain keratin or other proteins, such as beer and egg; manufacturers claim that these additives replace the protein lost in dry or damaged hair. According to the American Medical Association, there is little evidence to substantiate this claim. If these proteins do have an effect, it is similar to the coating effect of other conditioners.

Using Oils and Additives

Even if the arsenal of additives used by commercial soapmakers were readily available to the home soapmaker, most home crafters would still turn to simple, natural alternatives. The Additives Guide below should offer you plenty of options for shampoo "fillers," but don't stop there — all crafts should be approached in a spirit of adventure and experiment.

 GREAT SHAMPOO ADDITIVES

See page 42 for more information, but here's a brief recap of some excellent shampoo additives.

▶ BORAX. An excellent emulsifier, detergent, lather stabilizer, and thickening agent. One research source claims that extended use of borax can dry hair; another source claims that borax moisturizes. The best bet for home soapmakers is to try it for themselves.

▶ CASTOR OIL. A superb cleanser as well as a conditioner and moisturizer.

▶ ESSENTIAL OILS. Lavender, rosemary, and clary sage are herbs that purportedly condition hair and stimulate hair growth.

▶ GLYCERIN. One or 2 ounces added to a pound of shampoo is an excellent moisturizer and conditioner, creating shiny, lustrous hair.

▶ OLIVE OIL. Though all the formulations in this book offer the soapmaker a choice of soft oils, special attention should be paid to olive oil in formulating shampoos. Because of its molecular structure, olive oil is extremely gentle and moisturizing. Sweet almond oil also shares these virtues.

▶ SULFONATED CASTOR OIL. As a superfatting agent, 2 to 3 teaspoons sulfonated castor oil per 1 pound of shampoo adds richness and emollience without compromising the clarity of the liquid.

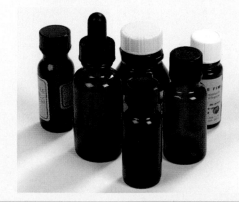

---

shampoo formulations

This section includes a wide variety of shampoo formulations, all based on the step-by-step instructions in chapter 2. If you have dry hair, look for formulations lower in coconut oil and higher in soft oils, castor oil, lanolin, jojoba, and cocoa butter. The addition of glycerin and/or sulfonated castor oil to the shampoo will moisturize and condition.

You can also formulate your own shampoo. Oily hair will benefit from shampoos high in coconut oil and lower in soft oils.

Unless otherwise directed, follow the instructions for mixing and cooking in chapter 2. You'll need soft oil — such as olive, almond, canola, safflower, or soy — for most of these recipes. Two rules apply to all of the recipes in this chapter:

If you're using the alcohol/lye method to make your soap, add 20 ounces of ethanol or iso-propyl alcohol to the oil and lye solution.

To neutralize the soap, add 4½ ounces of a 20 percent boric or citric acid solution or 4½ ounces of a 33 percent borax solution. *Note:* If you use borax as an emulsifier or thickener, no neutralizers will be necessary.

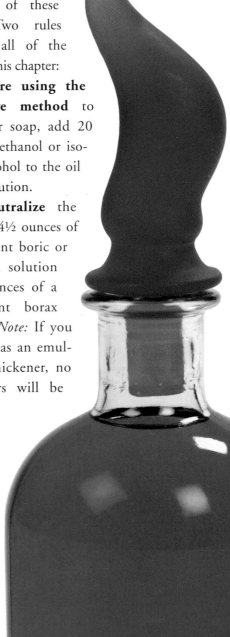

Basic Shampoo

This simple-to-make shampoo is high-foaming and has enough soft oil for emollience.

Oils
37 ounces coconut oil
11 ounces soft oil of choice

Lye solution
13 ounces potassium hydroxide
39 ounces soft or distilled water

▶ **You can use the same dyes to color shampoos and other liquid soaps; try blending custom shades.**

Castor Oil–Coconut Oil Shampoo

Castor oil conditions, moisturizes, and cleanses.

Oils

    39 ounces coconut oil
    8 ounces castor oil

Lye solution

    13 ounces potassium hydroxide
    39 ounces soft or distilled water

Vitamin E Hair Booster

A moisturizing formula, this shampoo contains vitamin E.

Oils

    42 ounces coconut oil
    3 ounces wheat germ oil
    3 ounces jojoba

Lye solution

    13 ounces potassium hydroxide
    39 ounces soft or distilled water

Jojoba Conditioning Shampoo

Like lanolin, jojoba moisturizes and conditions. The additional castor oil makes this a very rich and conditioning shampoo.

Oils

    37 ounces coconut oil
    9 ounces castor oil
    4 ounces jojoba oil

Lye solution

    13 ounces potassium hydroxide
    39 ounces soft or distilled water

Gentle Shampoo

The high percentage of soft oils and rosin makes this a very mild shampoo.

Oils

    25 ounces coconut oil
    12 ounces soft oil of choice
    6 ounces castor oil
    5 ounces rosin

Lye solution

    12 ounces potassium hydroxide
    36 ounces soft or distilled water

Liquid Silk Shampoo

Lanolin, which is almost identical to the oil found on our own hair, conditions and moisturizes.

Oils

    32 ounces coconut oil
    12 ounces soft oil of choice
    3 ounces lanolin

Lye solution

    12 ounces potassium hydroxide
    36 ounces soft or distilled water

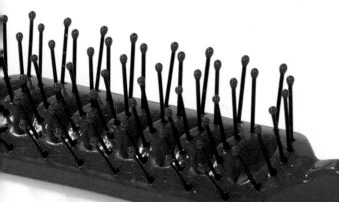

Revitalizing Rosin Shampoo

Rosin adds a rich, cold-cream finish to this shampoo.

Oils

- 37 ounces coconut oil
- 5 ounces soft oil
- 5 ounces rosin

Lye solution

- 13 ounces potassium hydroxide
- 39 ounces soft or distilled water

Goldilocks Shampoo

This is a shampoo high in vitamin E and moisturizers. The natural color of the wheat germ oil imparts a beautiful amber hue to the liquid.

Oils

- 34 ounces coconut oil
- 10 ounces wheat germ oil
- 6 ounces castor oil

Lye solution

- 13 ounces potassium hydroxide
- 39 ounces soft or distilled water

Marvelous Moisturizing Shampoo

High in castor oil and relatively low in coconut oil, this is an excellent shampoo for dry or dandruffy hair.

Oils

- 24 ounces coconut oil
- 13 ounces soft oil of choice
- 11 ounces castor oil
- 2 ounces lanolin

Lye solution

- 12 ounces potassium hydroxide
- 36 ounces soft or distilled water

Hawaiian Islands Shampoo

Cocoa butter, long used by the Hawaiians to condition the hair, is an excellent moisturizer.

Oils

- 35 ounces coconut oil
- 11 ounces soft oil of choice
- 2 ounces cocoa butter

Lye solution

- 13 ounces potassium hydroxide
- 39 ounces soft or distilled water

> Because rosin has a much higher melt point than oil, melt the rosin with 10 ounces of coconut oil. After the rosin has completely dissolved, add the remainder of the oils.

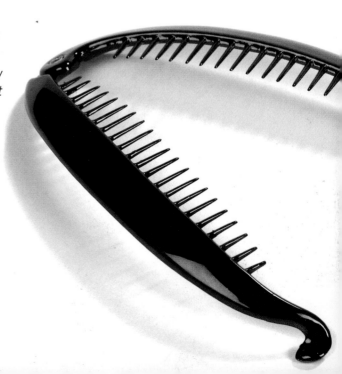

baby shampoos

"Old-fashioned" baby shampoos used by hospitals were formulated with nothing but olive oil and potassium hydroxide. Olive oil is composed of almost 90 per- cent oleic acid, an extremely mild fatty acid. As a base for soap, olive oil creates a gentle, moisturizing lather, making it ideal for a baby's sensitive skin.

100% Castile Soap Shampoo

Castile soap was originally a 100 per- cent olive oil soap, named for the Castile region in Spain. This type of soap makes the mildest of shampoos, ideal for baby's tender skin. It's not only for babies!

Oils
48 ounces olive oil

Lye solution
10 ounces potassium hydroxide
30 ounces soft or distilled water

For additional mildness, add 4 to 6 ounces of glycerin and 3 to 4 tablespoons of sulfon- ated castor oil to the recipes for 100% Castile Soap Shampoo and Sud- sy Fun Shampoo.

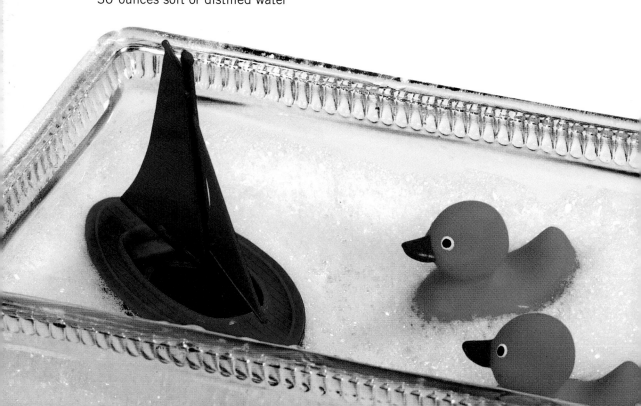

Sudsy Fun Shampoo

One hundred percent castile soap lacks a full lather. When 10 percent coconut oil is added, the soap remains mild but produces a better lather.

Oils
>   41 ounces olive oil
>   5 ounces coconut oil

Lye solution
>   10 ounces potassium hydroxide
>   30 ounces soft or distilled water

> One of the very first shampoos was soapless; it was based on sulfonated castor and olive oils.

▶ **You'll get peace of mind by formulating your own all-natural baby shampoos.**

"Soapless" Shampoo

At first, it's going to feel quite strange applying a latherless oil to the hair instead of soap. But you'll be pleasantly surprised — sulfonated castor oil makes a very decent shampoo.

>   1 cup sulfonated castor oil
>   1 tablespoon glycerin
>   1 tablespoon mineral or
>   baby oil
>   fragrance of choice

Mix together all ingredients, and stir for half a minute to homogenize. Because sulfonated castor oil is so soluble, no heating of the oils is necessary. Add fragrance. Use as you would a regular shampoo.

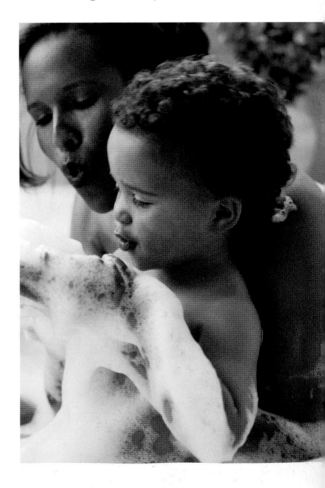

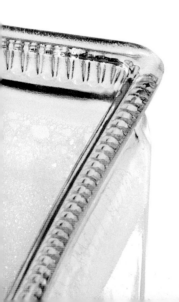

dog shampoos

As the saying goes, animals are people, too, and anything you lather with can be used to lather your pet. All the shampoo formulations in this chapter are suitable for dogs. If your dog has special problems, such as eczema, consider the mild 100% Castile Soap Shampoo or a formulation lower in coconut oil. You might also add glycerin and sulfonated castor oil to the shampoo for additional emollience.

▼ Essential oils, which are made from plants, are terrific additions to liquid soap blends.

Essential Oils for Flea Control

Lather aside, flea control is foremost on most dog owners' minds. For natural flea control, many essential oils possess fragrances particularly repellent to fleas; these oils include citronella, peppermint, lavender, rosemary, tea tree, cedarwood, rose geranium, cedar, clove, eucalyptus, pennyroyal, clary sage, and pine oils. Add 2 teaspoons (or more if desired) of essential oil to 1 pound of shampoo base, or try one of the blends below. *Note:* Essential oils are *not* insecticides.

Fresh-Scent Blend

1 part clove essential oil
1 part peppermint essential oil
1 part lemon essential oil

Herbal Flea Tamer

2 parts eucalyptus essential oil
1 part lavender essential oil
2 parts geranium essential oil
1 part cedarwood essential oil

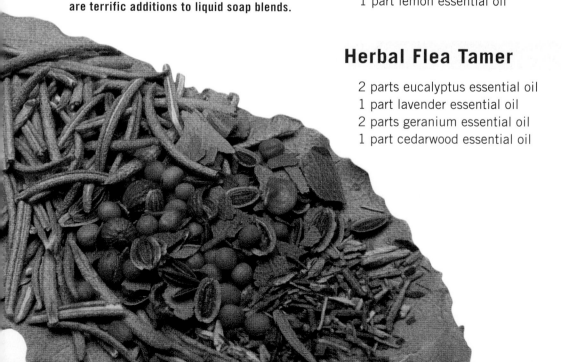

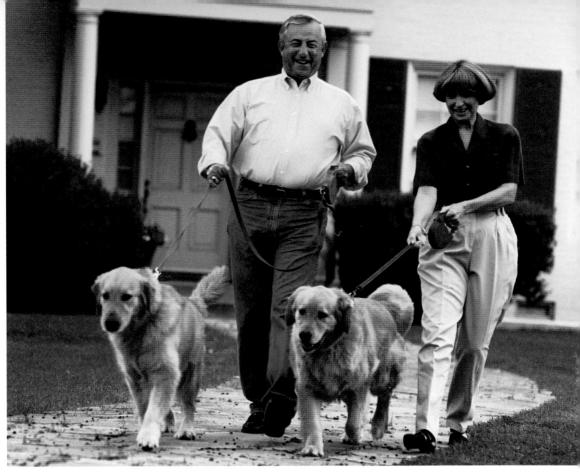

▲ Put the power of herbs to work in dog shampoos that help repel fleas, ticks, and other pests.

Pennyroyal–Citronella Special

5 parts pennyroyal essential oil
3 parts citronella essential oil

Minty Dog

1 part tea tree essential oil
1 part citronella essential oil
3 parts peppermint essential oil

Woodsy Blend

2 parts pine essential oil
1 part rosemary essential oil
1 part tea tree essential oil
6 parts orange essential oil

Great Outdoors

1 part lavender essential oil
2 parts cedarwood essential oil
1½ parts clove essential oil

Clean 'n' Green

1 part clary sage essential oil
2 parts peppermint essential oil
½ part eucalyptus essential oil

Lemon-Fresh Repellent

3 parts lemon essential oil
1 part citronella essential oil
1 part rosemary essential oil

sumptuous

(5) bath &

shower gels

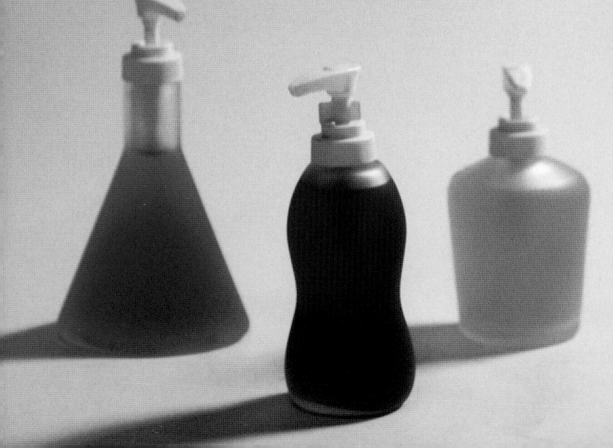

Viewed through a microscope, gels appear as fine, filamentous chains of soap molecules; these filamentous chains are what give gels their "elasticity."

Gels are "changelings." They exist in a very narrow window between liquid and semisolid, and you must do some fine-tuning to create that ideal proportion of soap to water. Slight excesses of water turn the gel into liquid soap; slight deficiencies of water make the gel revert to paste. Gels are also temperamental in regard to temperature. High temperatures thin gels; low temperatures congeal them.

Luckily for the home soapmaker, there are fairly simple solutions to the problems encountered in formulating these beautiful, though elusive, soaps.

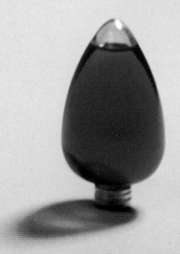

procedure for making gels

Use steps 1 through 7 of the paste method (on pages 22–27) for gel soap-making, then continue with the following steps. Don't use the alcohol/lye method to make gels; excess alcohol prevents gel from thickening.

Step 1: Add Solvents and Neutralizers

Cook the paste for 3 hours, remove the soap pot from the double boiler, and place it directly over medium heat on the stove. For every pound of paste, add 1 to 1½ ounces of alcohol and 4 ounces of glycerin. A 6-pound batch of soap will therefore require 6 to 9 ounces of alcohol

▼ Make bath and shower gels by first following the basic paste method.

and 24 ounces of glycerin. At this phase, you'll also add the neutralizing solution (borax, citric acid, or boric acid) at a rate of 4 tablespoons per 6 pounds of soap. If borax is to be used as an emulsifier or thickener, forgo the use of neutralizers.

Step 2: Cook

Stir the paste, alcohol, and glycerin together and cook until the paste is completely dissolved. If enough alcohol evaporates, the paste won't dissolve; in this case, add a few extra ounces of alcohol. After all the lumps have dissolved, stir in 6 ounces of distilled water per pound of paste, or 36 ounces of water for a full 6-pound recipe. Weigh the soap pot, then return the pot to the stove, and begin cooking. The solution is initially quite thin and, when stirred, produces a very billowy head of foam. After water and alcohol begin evaporating, the solution thickens. The foam thickens, too, becoming heavier and "creamier" as the bubbles condense.

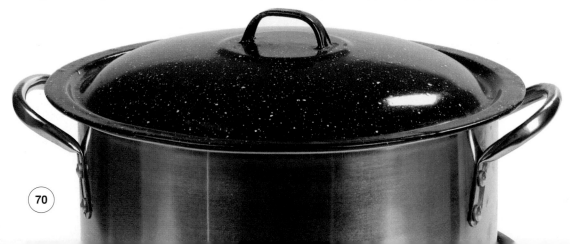

Step 3: Add Water

Reweigh the soap pot. By the time the foam becomes thick and creamy, approximately 12 to 16 ounces of water and alcohol will have evaporated from the soap stock. Scoop the foam to one side of the pot in order to view the soap solution. It will look noticeably different now; a thin, congealed crust will appear on the surface, and when swirled in the pot, the soap won't be completely fluid. Instead, it exhibits a "jiggly" and elastic behavior.

Step 4: Test the Viscosity

Remove the pot from the stove, and prepare a test sample of the stock by scooping up a teaspoon of solution (foam-free) and ladling it onto the top of an inverted quart jar. Cover the sample immediately with a piece of plastic wrap to prevent evaporation, then allow the sample to cool. To hasten cooling, chill the jar by placing it in the freezer for a few minutes.

If the cooled sample is watery, bring the soap back to a boil, and evaporate 2 to 3 more ounces of water. Test again. The state of "readiness" for a gel is partly subjective. Some soapmakers may desire a very thick liquid, while others may want a true gel, a concentration of approximately 45 to 50 percent soap.

Step 5: Add Dyes and Fragrances

Cook until the desired viscosity is achieved, then spoon off the foam, which can be diluted and used as a liquid soap base. Dye, fragrance, and bottle the finished gel immediately. If left to cool in the open air before bottling, gels develop a thick crust on the surface; these crusts are impossible to reincorporate into the solution. A small addition of borax will help emulsify the solution and prevent separation; use ½ ounce of 33 percent borax solution per pound of gel.

▼ Let your imagination go wild when you make color blends for your gels!

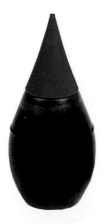
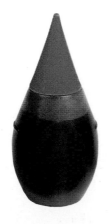
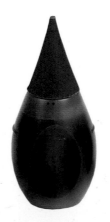
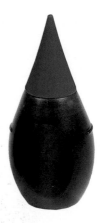

alternative gel-making method

Because borax works so well for thickening soft oil–based soaps, it's a perfect fit for gels that are always formulated with high proportions of soft oil.

If you wish to forgo the use of alcohol and glycerin, dissolve the paste in enough boiling water to bring all the soap into solution (1 to 2 pounds of water per pound of paste). Add 1 to 3 ounces of borax to the water at the same time you add the paste. The amount of borax you use depends upon how viscous you want the gel. This requires a little experimentation. You can always add more borax at any time during the cooking or even after the solution has cooled. (If you add extra borax during the cooking phase, dissolve it first in a little hot water.)

After the paste and borax have dissolved, create a stronger soap concentration by continuing to boil the solution. When the soap shows signs of thickening, test its viscosity by spooning out small samples onto a chilled, inverted glass. Cover the cooling samples with

▶ **Chill a glass or measuring cup before using it to test soap viscosity.**

plastic wrap to avoid further evaporation; this will give you a more accurate picture of the soap's consistency. Cook and sample frequently until the desired thickness is reached.

Because borax increases the viscosity of soft oil–based soaps, your soap will become a gel at a lower soap-to-water ratio than when you use the other gel method outlined on page 70. Because of the borax, no neutralizers will be necessary.

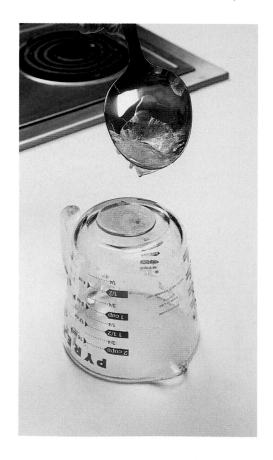

shower gel recipes

Gels have traditionally been formulated with high percentages of soft oils, which lend a smooth, salvelike pliancy to the finished soap. However, soft oils produce low lathers; one-half ounce of 33 percent borax solution per pound of gel will help improve the lather. The coconut oil in all the following formulations will also boost lather.

Follow the directions on pages 70–71 to make any of the recipes in this chapter. You'll need soft oil — such as olive, almond, canola, safflower, or soybean — for all these recipes. In addition, you'll want to neutralize the soap with 4½ ounces of a 20 percent boric or citric acid solution or 4½ ounces of a 33 percent borax solution. *Note:* If you use borax as an emulsifer or thickener, no neutralizers will be necessary.

Basic Shower Gel

This gel is very mild and emollient because of the high percentage of soft oils. Formulate with olive or almond oil to create an excellent "baby gel."

Oils
- 43 ounces soft oil of choice
- 5 ounces coconut oil

Lye solution
- 11 ounces potassium hydroxide
- 33 ounces soft or distilled water

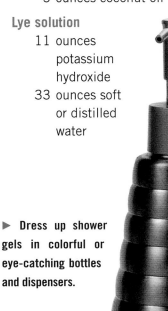

▶ **Dress up shower gels in colorful or eye-catching bottles and dispensers.**

Simple Coconut Oil Gel #1

This soap is mild like the Basic Shower Gel but a little foamier.

Oils
- 38 ounces soft oil of choice
- 7 ounces coconut oil

Lye solution
- 11 ounces potassium hydroxide
- 33 ounces soft or distilled water

Simple Coconut Oil Gel #2

Fairly high-foaming because of the high percentage of coconut oil, this gel is good for oily skin.

Oils
- 33 ounces soft oil of choice
- 14 ounces coconut oil

Lye solution
- 11 ounces potassium hydroxide
- 33 ounces soft or distilled water

 THE LANGUAGE OF SOAPMAKING

Old-time gel soapmakers possessed quite an interesting language to describe their soaps. Their texts are full of such phrases as "talking" soap, soaps that "audibly break into roses," and samples that "flower" when poured onto glass.

"Figged" soaps were specialty gels requiring care and experience on the part of the soapmaker. Oils high in stearic acid, such as palm oil or tallow, were blended into a gel base. Upon cooking and cooling, the stearic acid crystallized, forming a delicate lacelike pattern throughout the body of the gel. These "fig" formulations were described in such terms as "ricelike figging," "small, ryelike figging," or a "beautiful medium figging."

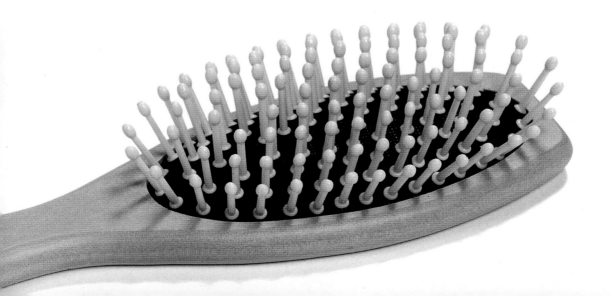

Coconut–Jojoba Fusion

The soft oils and jojoba make this gel ideal for dry skin or for preventing chapping in cold weather.

Oils

> 38 ounces soft oil of choice
> 3 ounces jojoba
> 9 ounces coconut oil

Lye solution

> 11 ounces potassium hydroxide
> 33 ounces soft or distilled water

Amber Allure

Rosin gives this gel a rich, cold-cream lather as well as a lovely nut-brown color.

Oils

> 34 ounces soft oil of choice
> 8 ounces coconut oil
> 7 ounces rosin

Lye solution

> 11 ounces potassium hydroxide
> 33 ounces soft or distilled water

Rich and Creamy Shower Gel

Palm oil (or tallow) lends this soap a little extra body.

Oils

> 28 ounces soft oil of choice
> 18 ounces coconut oil
> 4 ounces palm oil or tallow

Lye solution

> 12 ounces potassium hydroxide
> 36 ounces soft or distilled water

▼ **Boost the lather of shower gels by using netting sponges or loofahs.**

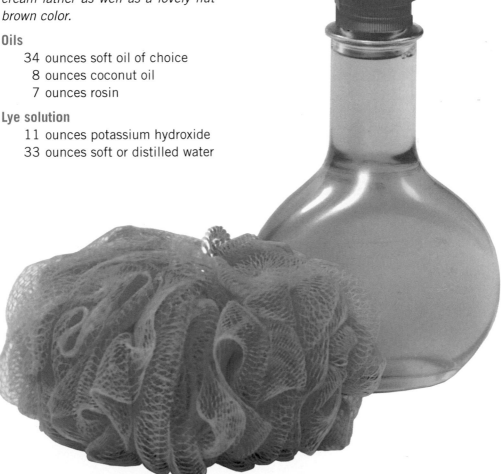

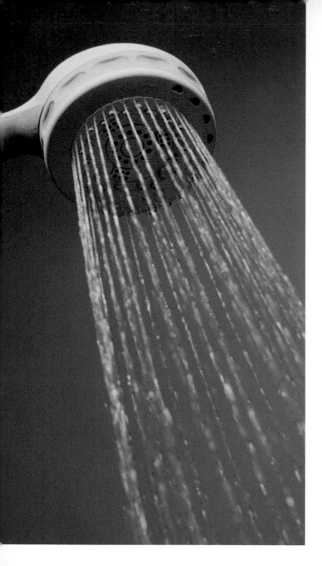

Coco-Loco Shower Gel

This is a high-foaming gel. Cocoa butter adds body and emollience.

Oils

24 ounces soft oil of choice
21 ounces coconut oil
3 ounces cocoa butter

Lye solution

12 ounces potassium hydroxide
36 ounces soft or distilled water

Summertime Smoothie

Try this very rich, mild, and soothing gel. Castor oil contributes to the clarity of the soap, offsetting the mild clouding caused by palm oil.

Oils

25 ounces soft oil of choice
9 ounces coconut oil
5 ounces palm oil
5 ounces castor oil

Lye solution

12 ounces potassium hydroxide
36 ounces soft or distilled water

Gels for Summertime

The higher the mercury in the thermometer climbs, the thinner gels become. One way to fortify gels against thinning is through additions of slight amounts of oils containing stearic and palmitic acids, whose higher melt points help prevent thinning. These oils need to be used sparingly because they cause clouding at higher percentages. To make any of these recipes, follow the instructions on pages 70–71.

A simple gel blended with a small percentage of alcohol served as an effective automobile soap in the early twentieth century.

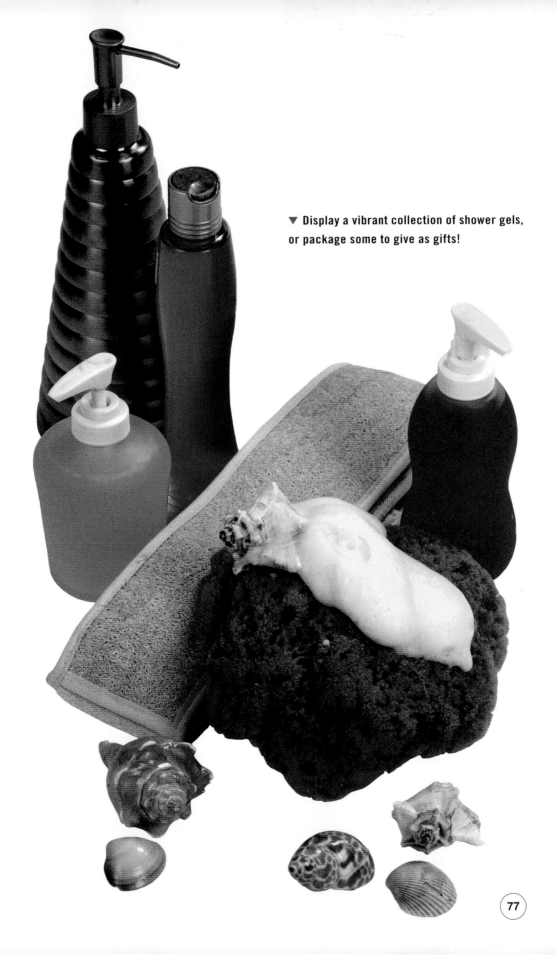

▼ Display a vibrant collection of shower gels, or package some to give as gifts!

luXurious
⑥ bubble
baths

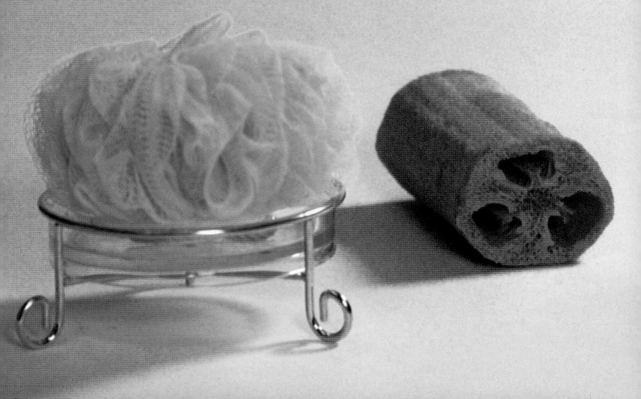

O f all soaps, either solid or liquid, bubble baths are most likely to be luxury items formulated almost exclusively for show. Getting these soaps to look their best with quick, high-foaming, long-lasting bubbles is a home soapmaker's prime consideration.

Following the guidelines given in this chapter, you'll be able to create rich and effective bubble baths. Of course, just because these bubble baths work well doesn't mean they can't look good too. Explore the possibilities in chapter 7, Dyeing & Fragrancing, which will show you how to make ordinary soap into something spectacular. As a bonus, I've included custom-made scents by professional soapmakers on pages 93 to 103; use these to transform your bathtime experience.

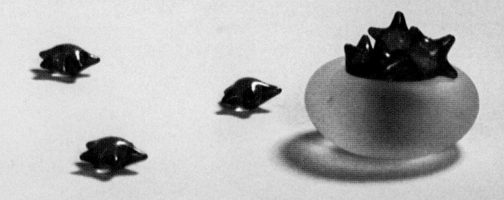

foam builders and stabilizers

Coconut oil (or any other oil high in lauric acid) forms the basis for all bubble baths because it produces the fastest, highest foam. Small amounts of soft oil can be added for emollience.

Soft oils high in oleic acid — such as olive, almond, and canola oils — create a higher, stabler lather than do soft oils composed of relatively little oleic acid.

Stabilizing the foam so that it persists in the bathtub is another big challenge. Commercial soapmakers have many chemicals at their disposal that home soapmakers lack. However, several additives mentioned in chapter 1 (glycerin, borax, and Calgon) work well as foam stabilizers.

If you wish to experiment first with the foaming action of these additives, dissolve 1 or 2 ounces of liquid soap in 10 to 12 ounces of water. Place the solution in a large pot, and whisk it for 20 seconds. Note how high and lasting the foam is. In a second pot, create an identical soap/water emulsion, then add a half teaspoon or so of whichever additive you're interested in. Whisk this for 20 seconds, and compare this foam with the nonadditive soap foam. In this manner, you can create your own bubble bath formulation.

▶ Lather will last longer if oils high in oleic acid are used in the recipe.

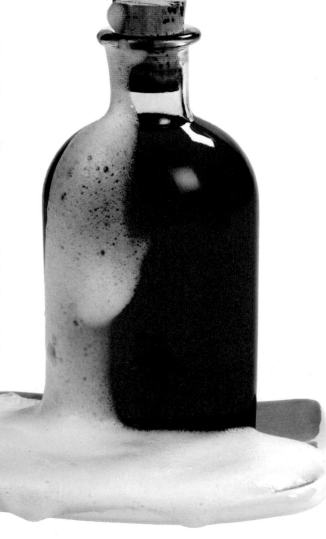

80

Glycerin

A few drops of glycerin added to ordinary dish soap creates an extraordinary bubble-blowing soap. The same principle can be applied to bubble bath formulations — a few ounces of glycerin added to the soap solution noticeably enhance foaming.

Borax

Borax (or Calgon) works even more effectively than glycerin. Borax acts as both a detergent and a foam stabilizer, making it one of the best extras for bubble bath formulations. In addition, borax is a water softener — a big plus if your bathwater is unsoftened.

Sodium– Potassium Soap

Sodium-based bar soaps markedly increase foaming when blended with a potassium soap.

Formulations combining sodium and potassium hydroxide are beyond the scope of this book because creating a homogenous emulsion with both hydroxides can be tricky on account of their differing solubilities. The emulsions tend to be grainy and very prone to separation. But for the first few bubble bath recipes, a few ounces of grated bar soap dissolved in hot potassium liquid soap will noticeably increase foaming. The sodium soap may cause a bit of clouding, however, particularly if the soap is superfatted. To avoid this problem, add the grated bar soap to the potassium-lye solution rather than after the potassium soap has cooked. Any excess fatty acids in the bar soap will be cooked and neutralized along with the potassium soap.

The sodium soap can be added to potassium soap in two different ways. First, you can add it as part of the potassium-lye solution. One big advantage of this method is that the presence of soap in the lye solution will increase the saponification rate by increasing emulsification of the oil and lye. If you wish to add 10 ounces of grated soap to your formulation, for example, dissolve it in 10 ounces of boiling water. Subtract this 10 ounces from the total amount of water needed for the lye solution. In a separate container, prepare the lye solution by mixing the hydroxide flakes with water (minus 10 ounces). After the soap has dissolved, add to the hot lye solution, then mix with the oils.

The grated soap can also be added after the potassium paste has been cooked and diluted. For every 1 ounce of soap, dissolve in 1 to 2 ounces of boiling water.

Powdered Milk

Milk is added to bath preparations as a soothing skin cleanser. Use a maximum of 4 percent milk (either dry buttermilk or regular nonfat) to the total diluted soap weight, or up to ⅔ ounce per pound of liquid soap.

Sulfonated Castor Oil

One other additive you might consider is sulfonated castor oil. Since it's completely water soluble, it can be used alone as a bath oil and blended with various essential oils, or it can be mixed into the bubble bath solution for added emollience.

Moisturizers, Foam Builders, and Stabilizers

Here are some guidelines for amounts of additives to use per pound of diluted soap base.

Additive	Amount
Glycerin	1 to 3 ounces
Borax*	1 to 3 teaspoons powder dissolved in 3 ounces hot water
Grated bar soap	2 to 8 ounces
Sulfonated castor oil	1 to 3 teaspoons
Powdered milk	up to ⅔ ounce

*Dry borax can also be added to the hot lye solution. As an emulsifier, it will speed saponification.

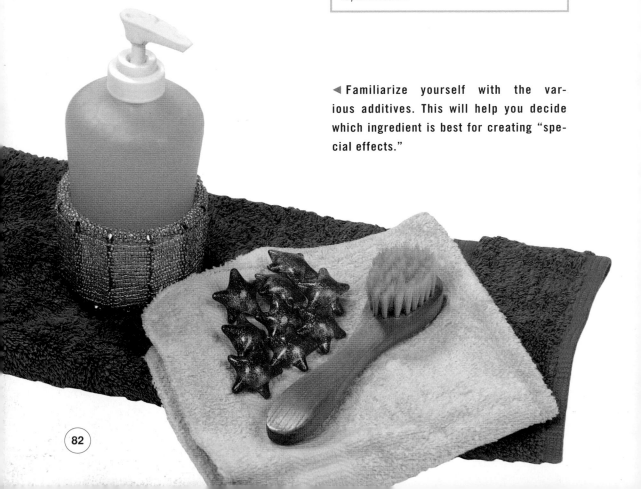

◄ Familiarize yourself with the various additives. This will help you decide which ingredient is best for creating "special effects."

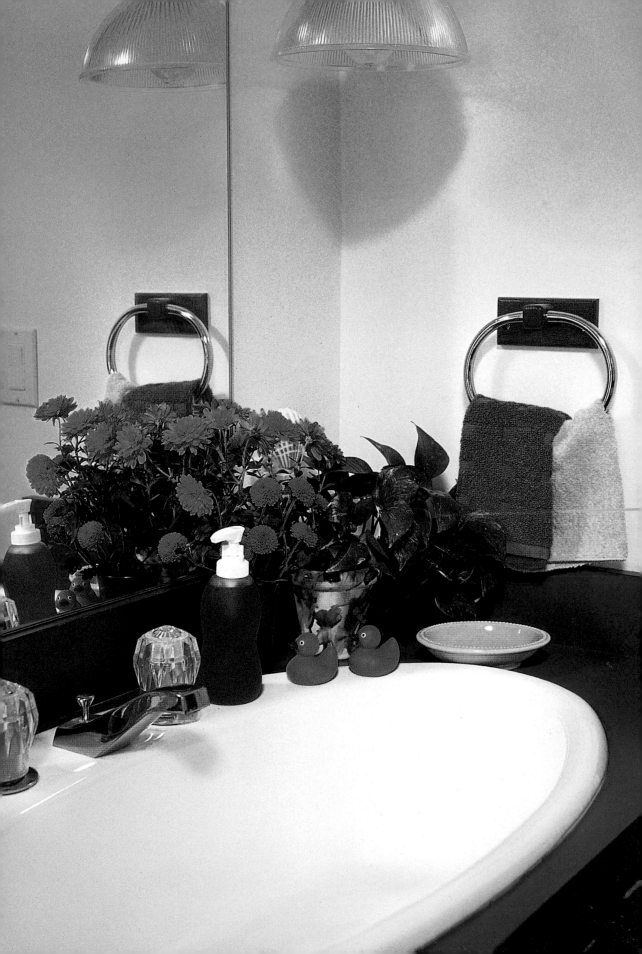

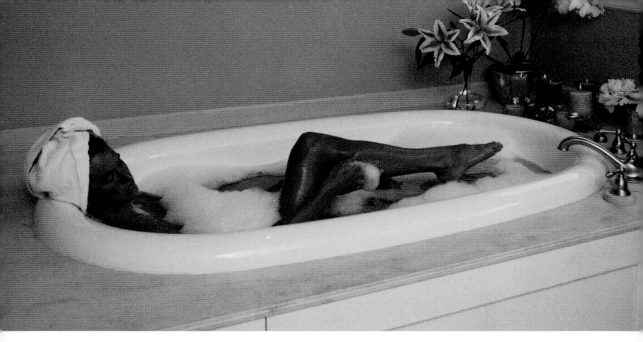

▲ A soothing bubble bath is only a few steps away with these simple formulas.

luxurious bubble bath recipes

At the end of the day, nothing is more relaxing than a hot bubble bath. Additives such as glycerin, sulfonated castor oil, and milk will enhance these soothing sensations, but consider too the aromatherapeutic effects of certain essential oils. For instance, the scent of rosemary helps relieve headaches, and lavender relaxes muscles. Or try adding some flower waters, such as rose water or orange water, directly to your bathwater.

Unless otherwise noted, follow the step-by-step instructions for making liquid soaps in chapter 2. Two special rules apply to all the recipes in this chapter:

If using the alcohol/lye method to make your soap, add 20 ounces ethanol or isopropyl alcohol to the oil and lye solution.

To neutralize the soap, add 4½ ounces of a 20 percent boric or citric acid solution or 4½ ounces of a 33 percent borax solution. *Note:* If you use borax as an emulsifer or thickener, no neutralizers will be necessary.

For higher, stabler foam, add borax, grated sodium soap, and/or glycerin according to the instructions on page 80.

Pure Coconut Oil Bubble Bath

This bath formula is very high foaming, but it may be somewhat drying to sensitive skin.

Oil
> 48 ounces coconut oil

Lye solution
> 14 ounces potassium hydroxide
> 42 ounces soft or distilled water

Cleopatra's Milk Bath

Legend says that Cleopatra took all-milk baths. Add sulfonated castor oil to the milk for extra mildness and emollience. After neutralizing and diluting the entire batch of paste, add the sulfonated castor oil and powdered milk (dissolved in hot water). Mix well into bubble bath.

Oils
> 44 ounces coconut oil
> 5 ounces olive, canola, or
>   almond oil

Lye solution
> 14 ounces potassium hydroxide
> 42 ounces soft or distilled water

Moisturizers
> ½ cup sulfonated castor oil
> 1 cup powdered milk

▶ **Why buy store brands when you can make bubble bath that is custom-tailored to your skin's needs?**

Olive Oil Bubble Bath

Olive oil not only adds emollience but foams well, too.

Oils
> 36 ounces coconut oil
> 12 ounces olive oil

Lye solution
> 13 ounces potassium hydroxide
> 39 ounces soft or distilled water

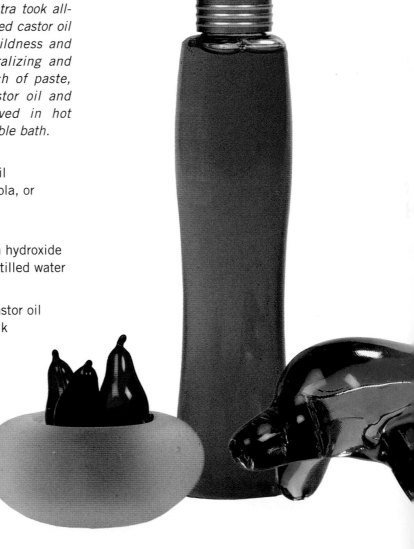

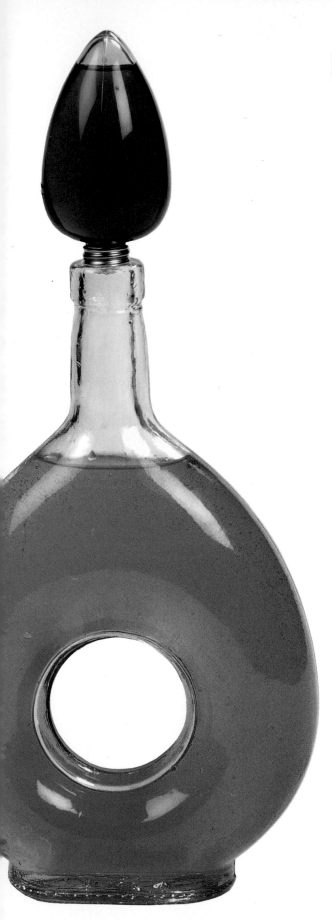

Supersudsy Bubble Bath

Adding sodium soaps to a potassium base is one of the best ways to enhance and prolong bubble bath foam.

Oils

42 ounces coconut oil

8 ounces olive, canola, or almond oil

Lye solution

14 ounces potassium hydroxide

20 ounces soft or distilled water

Foam Stabilizer

22 ounces grated sodium soap

Special instructions: The following variation applies to the basic instructions outlined in chapter 2.

1. Dissolve the potassium hydroxide in 20 ounces of water. (The potassium hydroxide actually requires a total of 42 ounces of water, but the remaining 22 ounces will be used to create a soap solution.) Bring the remaining 22 ounces of water to a boil, and add grated sodium soap; cover and cook at a gentle boil until the soap has dissolved. A few ounces of alcohol added to the solution aids in dissolving the soap.

2. Now mix the soap solution with the lye solution, and stir into the hot oils. Besides enhancing foam, the soap accelerates saponification.

◀ **Never underestimate the power of great presentation: This gorgeous bottle makes a statement of its own.**

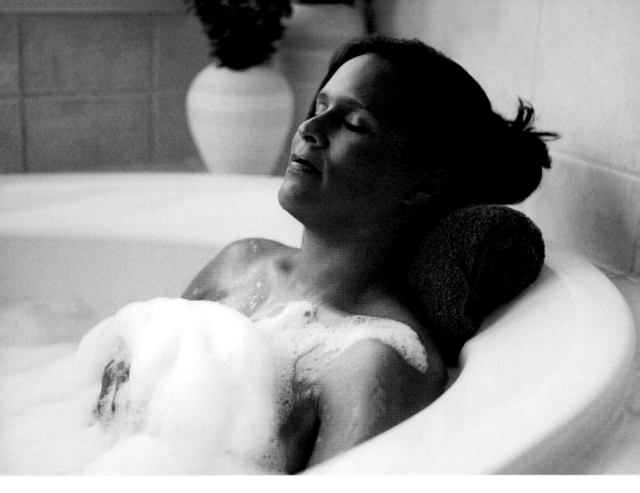

Essence of Rosin Bubble Bath

One turn-of-the-century formulary claimed that soap for bubble blowing could be improved with a mixture of soap and rosin. Try it in your bubble bath! Besides increasing foam and emollience, the rosin imparts a wonderful earthy fragrance to the bath. You may need no additional fragrances.

Oils

    40 ounces coconut oil
     5 ounces olive, canola, or
       almond oil
     8 ounces rosin

Lye solution

    14 ounces potassium hydroxide
    42 ounces soft or distilled water

▲ Make up several different bubble baths, and choose your favorite by taking each for a "test drive"!

> Rosin has a high melt point and burns easily. Melt it over a double boiler with part or all of the olive and coconut oils until dissolved.

dyeing
7
&
fragrancing

rose is a rose is a rose." Or so said Gertrude Stein. Many people have puzzled over the meaning of this phrase, but who knows — perhaps she was referring to hot-process soapmaking, in which the fragrance rose and the color rose both remain rose after being added to soap.

Not so with cold-process soapmaking, where there is much trial and error. Colors and scents are added before the soap is neutral, so the additives must pass through a brutal rite of passage in which they're subjected to extremely high levels of alkali. Some make it out alive, but many don't. All cold-process soapmakers have experienced the amazing vanishing scent, or the blue color turned dishwater gray.

Hot-process soapmaking will come as a welcome relief. There's no second-guessing the soap and how it will affect colors and scents, because the soap is neutral and has lost its "teeth." You get to be selfish, thinking only about your own wants and needs!

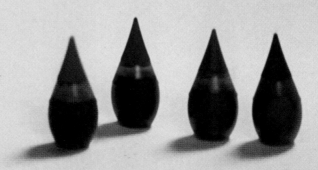

dyes
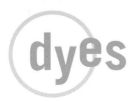

Most of the soap formulations in this book will yield soaps in a color range of pale gold to deep amber, depending on the base oils. You may not want to alter these lovely colors with additional dye. If dye is used, always proceed conservatively with just a few drops at a time. It's very easy to color a liquid soap too much.

Food Coloring

Food-grade dyes from the supermarket are the simplest and easiest to start with. Blue, green, red, and yellow remain stable in liquid soap. Food dyes come in both liquid and gel form; when using gels, be sure to dissolve the dye in hot water before adding it to your soap. If the dye is added directly to the soap, you can't really anticipate how saturated the final color will be because the gel takes some time to dissolve.

▶ **Use a single color, or create subtle variations by blending two or more dyes.**

Soap Dyes

Food dyes can be blended to create other colors: blue and yellow for turquoise, red and yellow for orange. The color combinations are a bit limited, however, because of the limitations in the shades of the four colors themselves. There's a bit too much yellow in both the red and the blue, for example, to yield a decent purple. Luckily, various colors of soap dyes are readily available. Resources has an extensive list of soap dye suppliers.

Fabric dyes are not recommended for soapmaking because they contain salt, which will cloud liquid soaps and gels.

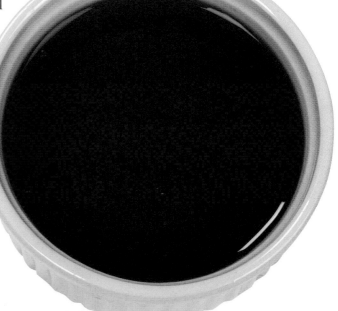

fragrances

Fragrances, like dyes, remain true to form when added to hot-processed soap. The lovely, captivating fragrance you bought last week is the same one you'll smell when opening your bottle of homemade gel or shampoo.

The fruity fragrances in particular can never be duplicated with essential oils. Hot-process soaps are an ideal vehicle for these fruity notes, but these scents usually lose much of their "color" and "brightness" when added to cold-process soaps.

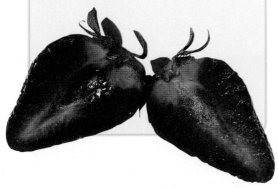

Fragrance Oils

There are two ways to fragrance: by using synthetic, laboratory-produced scents or by using true essential oils derived from plant sources. These distinctions aren't quite as black and white as they seem on the surface, because most "synthetics" are a blend of both essential and synthetic aromas. These blends can contain scores of different oils and compounds. One of the great benefits of synthetic fragrances is that the amateur soapmaker can enjoy the fruits of much trial-and-error blending done by the artists who work for fragrance companies.

Another advantage of using fragrance oils is the wide range of choices they offer the home soapmaker, not only in terms of price but also in terms of novelty. A pound of true essential oil of rose or jasmine can cost $2,000 or more. A good synthetic jasmine can be purchased for $20 to $40 a pound. And there is no true essential oil of strawberry, pear, or dewberry.

For fragrance oil suppliers, please see Resources.

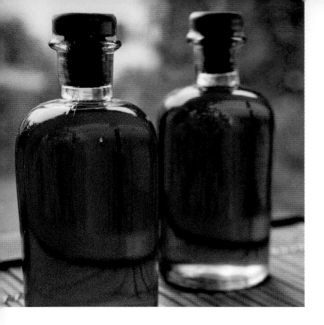

Pure Essential Oils

What pure essential oils lack in novelty they make up for in romance. Most essential oils come from very exotic places — deep forests in Indonesia or China, sun-drenched hills in the south of France. You can't help but think about these places when you open a bottle of essential oil, nor can you help but think about the people who produce them, often using centuries-old techniques, and then contemplate all the leaves, twigs, and flowers required to produce these oils. For instance, thousands of pounds of petals are needed to yield 1 pound of rose oil.

▼ You'll find pure essential oils and even fragrance oils that smell like fresh plants and spices.

Essential oils have been distilled from plants for centuries, and the art of perfuming goes back just as far. The blending of essential oils to create the right "notes" and effects is one of the most interesting and creative aspects of home soapmaking. Hours and hours can go into getting just the right scent, and like a feel for any art, a certain feel for fragrancing comes with time and experience.

There's some controversy over whether essential oils are healthier for the skin than fragrance oils. It's easy to reflexively state that "natural is always better than synthetic," but some essential oils, such as cinnamon, can cause extreme allergic skin reactions. It all comes down to personal preference. One advantage essential oils have over fragrance oils, however, is their aromatherapeutic value in relaxing, stimulating, or altering moods.

Leftover shavings from pencil manufacture are distilled into essential oil of cedarwood.

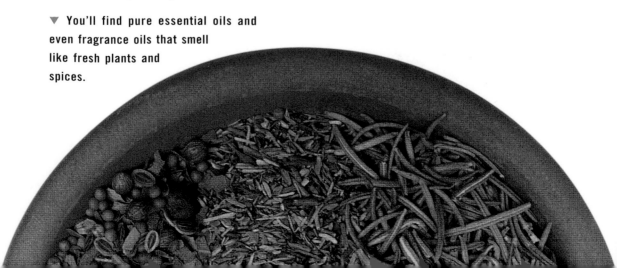

fragrance formulations

The art of soapmaking is now experiencing an incredible revival, and along with that, the art of fragrancing is also gaining renewed interest. Thousands of amateur soapmakers and small-scale soapmaking businesses now create their own unique fragrance blends. The blends in this chapter (both pure essential oils and fragrance oils) have all been created by small-scale soap-business owners across the country. All these businesses gladly sell to the mail-order public. See Resources for more information.

Most commercial soaps are fragranced at a 1 percent rate, or 1 percent of fragrance per weight of the soap. But fragrancing is very subjective, and some fragrances are much stronger than others. Use this as a rough guideline only.

Naturally Wild for Men

This blend is from Kathy Tarbox, a.k.a. The Petal Pusher, in Stanwood, Washington.

- 5 parts Swiss pine essential oil
- 3 parts clary sage essential oil
- 2 parts grapefruit essential oil
- 1 part lemongrass essential oil
- 1 part sandalwood essential oil

Sweet Harmony for Women

Another one of Kathy Tarbox's fabulous scents.

- 2 parts lemon verbena essential oil
- 2 parts jasmine essential oil
- 5 parts grapefruit essential oil
- 3 parts tuberose essential oil
- 3 parts bergamot essential oil
- 2 parts oakmoss essential oil

▶ **Grapefruit is an easily recognizable yet versatile fragrance that can be used in a number of soap blends.**

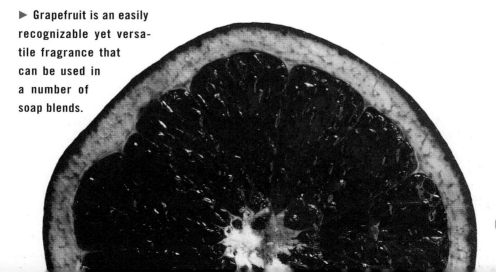

Smooth Operator

Renee Thompson of Country Scent-uals in Newalla, Oklahoma describes this recipe as "a sultry, mellow blend."

2 parts lavender essential oil
1 part ylang-ylang essential oil

SOAPMAKING HISTORY

British soapmakers had a particularly difficult time during the Middle Ages. The small soapmaking communities that developed around London were taxed on all the soap they produced. This tax rose so high that soapmaking kettles were fitted with lids that could be locked up by the tax collectors every night. This ensured that no illegal soap was manufactured under the cover of darkness.

Indian Dream

"The medicinal properties are what caused me to put [these oils] together," says Renee Thompson. "Even those who aren't happy with patchouli love this."

1 part sandalwood essential oil
1 part patchouli essential oil
4 parts sweet grass essential oil

Summer Fun

Another of Renee's blends, one she says is "very Beach Boys, summer, and fun."

2 parts mango fragrance oil
1 part pineapple fragrance oil
1 part coconut fragrance oil
1 part banana fragrance oil

Spring Scent

From Trisha Walton of Homesong Handcrafted Soaps, in Williamston, Michigan, comes this airy fragrance.

11 parts peach fragrance oil
8 parts grapefruit fragrance oil
1 part amber fragrance oil

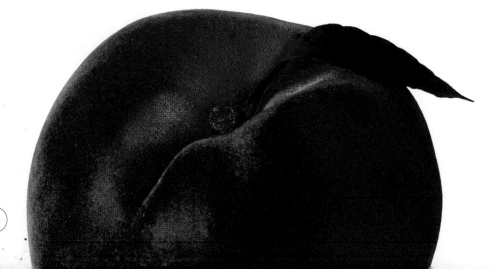

Citrus Refresher

Helen Dubovik of Blue Moon Botanicals in Kingston, Illinois, created this blend, which she describes as "a crisp and clean scent . . . mentally and creatively stimulating."

- 1 part bergamot essential oil
- 1 part grapefruit (preferably pink) essential oil

Love Potion #7

This is one of Helen Dubovik's romantic, exotic fragrances.

- 3 parts Bulgarian rose essential oil
- 2 parts sandalwood essential oil
- ¼ part ylang-ylang essential oil
- ⅛ part vanilla essential oil
- ¹⁄₁₆ part black pepper essential oil
- ¹⁄₁₆ part nutmeg essential oil

Sweet Earth

Says Helen, "[This scent is] warm and earthy [and] holds well in soap."

- 3 parts sandalwood essential oil
- 1 part patchouli essential oil
- 1 part lemon essential oil

3 Cs Soap Blend

Jill Sidney of Iowa Natural Soapworks in Davenport, Iowa, created this unique fragrance.

- 3 parts rose geranium essential oil
- 2½ parts palmarosa essential oil
- 2 parts rosewood essential oil
- 1 part basil essential oil

Mist Pine Barrens Soap Blend

Bob McDaniel of The Loom Rat in Chalfont, Pennsylvania, contributed this original blend.

- 1½ part white pine essential oil
- 1 part cypress essential oil
- 1 part cedarwood essential oil
- ¼ part guaiacwood essential oil

Meadow Garden

Also one of Jill Sidney's blends, this scent is simple yet beautiful.

- 3 parts rose fragrance oil
- 1 part clary sage essential oil

◄ ▼ **Fruity scents are very popular in soaps. Experiment with different types to find your favorites.**

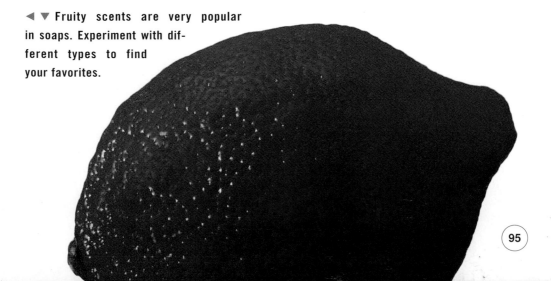

Citrus Delight

From Sharon Dodge of Serenity Soaps and Herb Gardens in Camano Island, Washington, comes this fruity fragrance that is "yummy enough to eat."

- 2 parts sweet orange essential oil
- 1 part lime essential oil
- 1 part pink grapefruit essential oil

Christmas Evergreen

Sharon Dodge also created this wonderful holiday scent.

- 2 parts pine essential oil
- 1 part cedarwood essential oil
- 1 part hemlock essential oil

Sultry Nights

A "warm-bodied scent for summer," this blend was contributed by Diana Johnson of Cat's Paw Enterprises in Port Townsend, Washington.

- 9 parts rose essential oil
- 5 parts clove essential oil
- 4 parts peppermint essential oil

Essential oil of orange comes from Haiti, compliments of Christopher Columbus. After discovering the New World, Columbus returned to Spain, bringing along the seeds of many different plants. Among these plants were the true bitter orange and the true sweet orange.

My Guy's Blend

Diana Johnson created this fragrance especially for guys.

- 10 parts caraway essential oil
- 5 parts lavender essential oil
- 3 parts rosemary essential oil

▼ **Rosemary and other piney fragrances are good choices when making soap blends for men.**

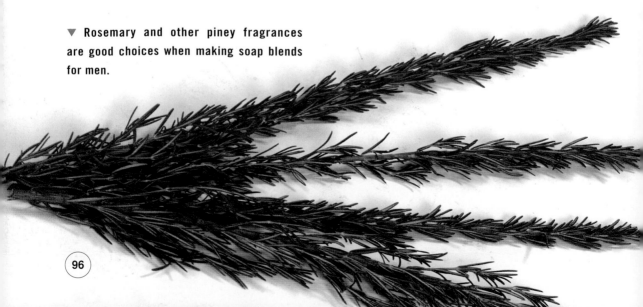

Patchouli–Almond Spice

This spicy blend is courtesy of Mary Byerly of Gentler Thymes Soap Company in Palos Heights, Illinois.

- 3 parts patchouli essential oil
- 2 parts bitter almond essential oil
- 1 part cassia essential oil

Bath Balm

This is another of Mary's creations. Lavender eases tired muscles, making it perfect for adding to a bubble bath soap.

- 20 parts lavender essential oil
- 4 parts tea tree essential oil
- 2 parts lemongrass essential oil
- 1 part cassia essential oil

Lemon Refresher

A "wake-up" blend from Mary Byerly.

- 12 parts lemon essential oil
- 4 parts bergamot essential oil
- 2 parts eucalyptus essential oil
- 1 part lavender essential oil

Classical Romance

A woodsy and exotic blend, courtesy of Mary Byerly.

- 2 parts ylang ylang essential oil
- 1 part rosewood essential oil

▶ Color and fragrance will transform common liquid soap into an exceptional treat.

Summer Garden

A flowery, sweet scent with some nice top notes of citrus, compliments of Gentler Thymes.

- 4 parts geranium essential oil
- 3 parts spearmint essential oil
- 2 parts sweet orange essential oil
- 2 parts grapefruit essential oil
- 1 part linden blossom essential oil

Sunshine Spirit

Karen White of Natural Impulse Handmade Soap and Sundries in Birmingham, Alabama, created this uplifting fragrance.

- 10 parts sweet orange essential oil
- 13 parts palmarosa essential oil
- 1 part *Litsea cubeba* essential oil

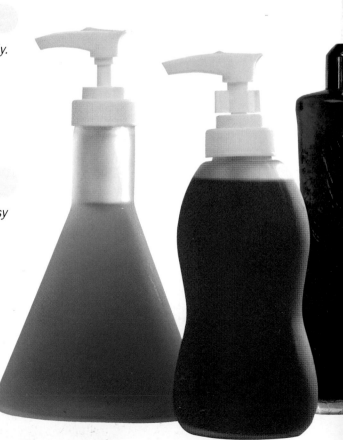

Island Breeze

Flowery with a hint of spice, this fragrance would go well in a summer gel. Compliments of Karen White.

- 2 parts jasmine, either essential oil or fragrance oil
- 1 part coriander essential oil

Honey Pie

Sweet and simple, this scent is compliments of Karen White.

- 1 part vanilla fragrance oil
- 1 part honey fragrance oil

Mint Julep

Another summery blend created by Karen White, this fragrance combines essential and fragrance oils.

- 8 parts honey fragrance oil
- 7 parts *Litsea cubeba* essential oil
- 4 parts peppermint essential oil
- 3 parts spearmint essential oil
- 3 parts heather fragrance oil

Too Sexy (Hers)

One more from Karen White — a mellow, "autumnal" blend.

- 4 parts pumpkin-pie spice fragrance oil
- 3 parts lavender essential oil

Dream Weaver

From Debbie Graybeal of Indian River Creations in Melbourne, Florida, comes this simple blend.

- 1 part clary sage essential oil
- 2 parts cedarwood essential oil
- 2 parts petitgrain essential oil

Flower Child

Flower Child is a warm, earthy blend from Indian River Creations.

- 1 part patchouli essential oil
- 2 parts *Litsea cubeba* essential oil
- 2 parts ginger essential oil

▶ **Don't stop at fruity fragrances; try vegetable, flower, and herb scents, too.**

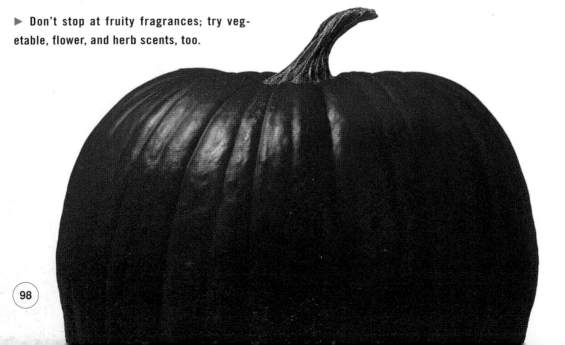

For Men

Reminiscent of a refreshing after-shave, this formula is from Debbie Graybeal.

- 2 parts tangerine essential oil
- 2 parts petitgrain essential oil
- 1 part lavender essential oil
- 1 part coriander essential oil
- ½ part cassia or cinnamon essential oil

Heavenly

A bracing concoction from Debbie — good for a "wake-up" shower gel.

- 1 part clove essential oil
- 1 part lavender essential oil
- 2 parts tangerine essential oil
- 2 parts grapefruit essential oil
- 2 parts lime essential oil
- 2 parts petitgrain essential oil
- 4 parts lemon essential oil

Tangerine Dream

One of Debbie's favorites, this is an excellent fragrance for a soothing bubble bath.

- 1 part patchouli essential oil
- 2 parts tangerine essential oil
- 4 parts clary sage essential oil
- 8 parts lavender essential oil

Lavender–Patchouli Blend

Tammy Hawk of the Southern Soap Company in Fultondale, Alabama, offers this blend.

- 1 part patchouli essential oil
- 3 parts lavender essential oil
- ¼ part cedarwood essential oil

CREATIVE MARKETING

Thomas Barratt, the "father of modern advertising," was a soapmaker. The son-in-law of Andrew Pears, Barratt made Pears soap into an internationally recognized brand with a series of bold and imaginative marketing techniques. He imported a quarter of a million French centimes and stamped one side with the name "Pears." These went into wide circulation before Parliament created a special law prohibiting the coins. Barratt was also the first person to reproduce fine art in poster form for the general populace.

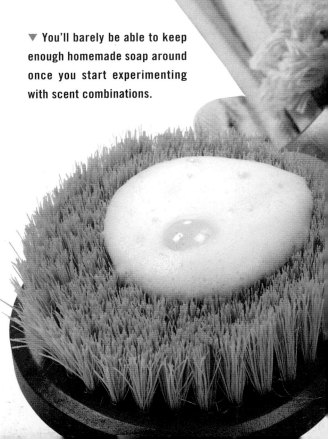

▼ You'll barely be able to keep enough homemade soap around once you start experimenting with scent combinations.

Eau de Cologne

This perfumelike fragrance is by Rebecca Keifer of the Delaware City Soap Company in Delaware City, Delaware.

- 4 parts sweet orange essential oil
- 3 parts lavender essential oil
- 3 parts rosemary essential oil
- 2 parts lemon essential oil

Rebecca's Patchouli

Rebecca Keifer also formulated this variation on a familiar favorite.

- 8 parts cedarwood essential oil
- 3 parts patchouli essential oil
- 3 parts geranium essential oil
- 1 part sassafras essential oil

Lime Smoothie

Lisa and Matt Redman of Flower Moon Soaps in Chestertown, Maryland, came up with this fun and fruity blend.

- 2 parts vanilla essential oil
- 2 parts Mexican lime essential oil

Old Kent Garden

Another blend courtesy of Lisa and Matt Redman, this scent recalls Victorian gardens.

- 1 part French lavender essential oil
- ½ part rosemary essential oil
- 1 part lemon verbena essential oil
- ½ part sweet basil essential oil
- 1 part rose essential oil

◄ **You can't go wrong with classic fragrances, such as rose, lavender, and patchouli.**

Rose of Bengal

This is another of Rebecca Keifer's special creations.

- 8 parts palmarosa essential oil
- 4 parts rosewood essential oil
- 1 part cinnamon leaf essential oil

Cinnamon Forest

This blend was provided by Maggie Anderson of Scentsables in Battle Ground, Washington.

- 4 parts cinnamon leaf essential oil
- 4 parts vanilla fragrance oil
- 2 parts patchouli essential oil
- 1 part lavender essential oil
- ½ part Peru balsam essential oil

Signature Blend of Squeaky Clean . . . Naturally!

From Darlene Nielsen of Squeaky Clean . . . Naturally! in Circleville, New York, comes this one-of-a-kind creation.

- 6 parts lavender essential oil
- 6 parts orange essential oil
- 4 parts ylang ylang essential oil
- 2 parts clary sage essential oil

Arabian Nights

Donna Ramsey of the Soap Box in Cochrane, Alberta, Canada, came up with this multilayered romantic blend.

- 2 parts rosewood essential oil
- 1 part patchouli essential oil
- 2 parts sandalwood essential oil
- 1 part neroli essential oil
- 1 part jasmine essential oil
- 1 part rose essential oil
- 2 parts white grapefruit essential oil
- 1 part bergamot essential oil
- 1 part gardenia essential oil

Tropical Citrus Blend

This is another of Donna Ramsey's trademark scents.

- 3 parts pink grapefruit essential oil
- 5 parts sweet orange essential oil
- 3 parts lemon essential oil
- 3 parts lime essential oil

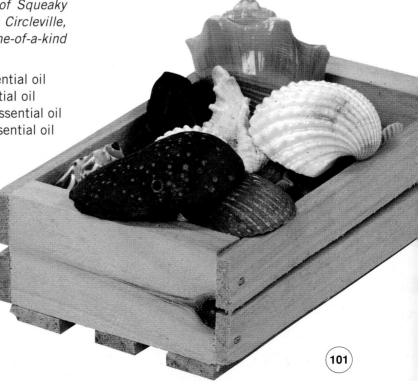

Lavender oil, made from a plant native to the Mediterranean region, is produced almost exclusively in southern France. Because it grows in relatively barren soils, it can spread like a weed. Early in the twentieth century, many marginal French farms were abandoned as the rural populace swarmed to the industrializing cities. Lavender moved in as the farmers moved out.

Strawberry–Rhubarb Pie

AnnaLiese Moran of Designs By AnnaLiese in Corvallis, Oregon, dreamed up this delicious scent.

   3 parts strawberry fragrance oil
   1 part rhubarb fragrance oil

Christmas Carnation

This spicy holiday fragrance was created by Bill and Trina Wallace of Snowdrift Farm Natural Products in Jefferson, Maine.

   1 part ylang ylang essential oil
   1 part clove bud essential oil

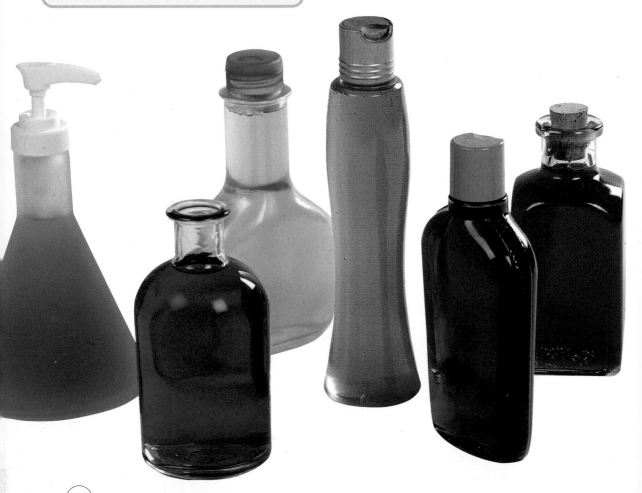

Noir Blend

Bill and Trina Wallace also concocted this mysterious scent.

   4 parts patchouli essential oil
   2 parts lavender essential oil
   1 part myrrh essential oil

Sea Breezy

Here's a terrific herbal blend, courtesy of Bill and Trina Wallace.

   2 parts *Eucalyptus citriodora* essential oil
   2 parts lemongrass essential oil
   1 part rosemary essential oil

Exotic Blend

Ethel Winslow of Pisces Rising Aromatherapy Arts and Crafts in Indianapolis, Indiana, created this inspired fragrance.

   6 parts ylang ylang essential oil
   2 parts black pepper essential oil
   2 parts coriander essential oil
   2 parts sweet orange essential oil

Sports Essential Blend

Ethel Winslow also formulated this blend with oils that help alleviate the pain of sports injuries. Peppermint relieves pain and stimulates circulation, eucalyptus relieves pain and warms muscles, marjoram relieves muscle spasms and warms the muscles, and lavender relieves pain and warms and balances muscles.

   1 part peppermint essential oil
   2 parts eucalyptus essential oil
   2 parts marjoram essential oil
   6 parts lavender essential oil

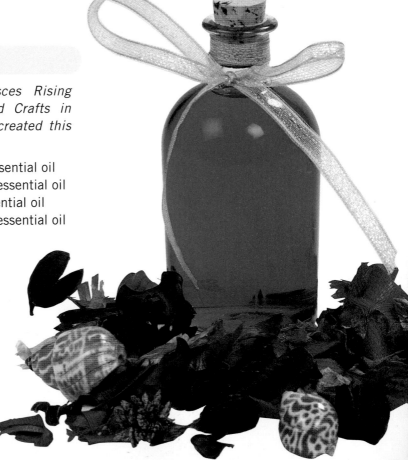

◄ **Choose fun containers, and wrap your creations with cellophane, paper, and bows for the perfect all-occasion gift.**

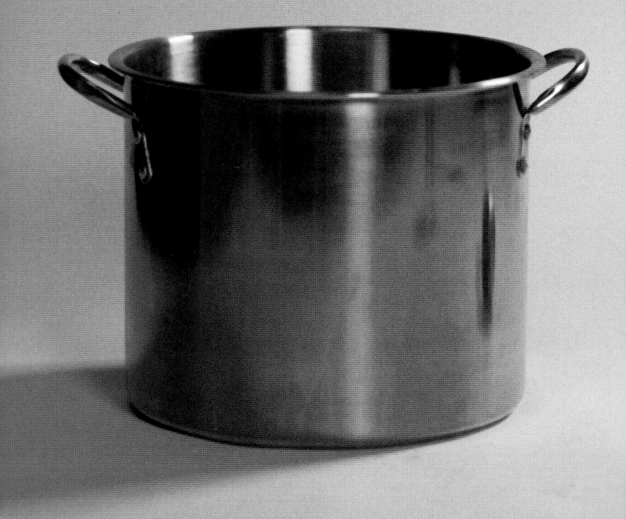

trouble-
⑧ shooting

inety-nine percent of all failures associated with liquid and gel soap-making are due to improper measurement of ingredients or undercooking of the soap stock. (An accurate scale and thermometer can save the home soapmaker much time and trouble.) The good news is that almost all these failures are correctable.

The first portion of this chapter presents many common liquid soap "ailments" along with simple suggestions for "cures." Some of these problems are associated with mismeasurement of oil or lye, however, and will require a little more attention. Imbalances in pH can be treated by the methods outlined in Correcting pH Problems on page 112.

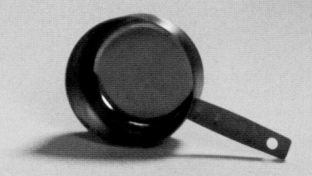

problems & solutions

Problem: Oil-lye emulsion doesn't thicken. Depending on the formulation and how you mix your ingredients, an emulsion should form within 15 minutes to an hour. If the emulsion hasn't thickened within an hour, your problem is due to understirring, low cooking temperatures, or incorrect measurement of ingredients.

Solution: If you've been mixing by hand with a spoon, switch to a stick blender, blender, or food processor. Also, make sure that your temperatures are in the 160 to 170°F (71 to 76°C) range. If these remedies don't work after another half hour of stirring, you've probably mismeasured your ingredients — most likely, the oils are in excess. Excess alkali usually manifests as a "curdled" appearance in the emulsion or else creates a "puffiness" that can't be stirred down. In the case of excess oils, consult Correcting Excess Fatty Acids on page 113.

Problem: Emulsion has a curdled appearance. This problem is occasionally caused by a wide disparity between the temperature of the oils and the lye solution before mixing. But most likely, it's due to excess alkali or insufficient oil. Strong lye solutions don't combine readily with oils, and a grainy, curdled appearance results.

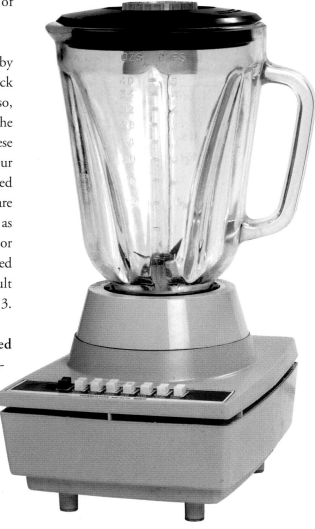

▶ Blending or stirring is one of the most important parts of soapmaking. Never skimp on this step.

Solution: If this problem was caused by wide temperature differences, add a few ounces of alcohol to the emulsion, and stir. The alcohol will help homogenize the emulsion, and it should smooth out within a few minutes. If your temperatures were correct, you have excess alkali. Refer to Correcting Excess Alkali on page 115 for further instructions.

Problem: Emulsion separates when cooking in double boiler. Potassium emulsions tend to "break" more easily than sodium emulsions. It's important to keep stirring the emulsion until it thickens to the consistency of saltwater taffy, then place it in the double boiler. In the case of soaps high in soft oils, such as gels, the emulsions won't be quite as sticky as those higher in coconut oil. Thinner emulsions may appear homogenous, but appearances can be deceptive.

> Regardless of the type of problem you're trying to solve, you should still follow the ingredient-handling cautions outlined in chapter 2.

Solution: Separated emulsions often require just a few more minutes of stirring with a hand blender to thicken properly.

Problem: Paste "puffs up" when cooking. Some amount of puffing is normal when the paste method is used. During the mixing phase, soap captures air, which then expands when heated.

Solution: Stirring with a spoon or spatula allows the air to escape. You may need to repeat this process a few more times in the next hour to hour and a half of cooking. Beyond that time, excessive puffing that doesn't seem to stir down is a good indication of too much alkali. Remedy this problem using the technique outlined in Correcting Excess Alkali on page 115.

Problem: An oily layer floats on top of alcohol-lye solution. The alcohol, oils, and lye solution need to be thoroughly mixed before the pot is capped with plastic and cooked.

Solution: Mixing should take just a few minutes, but even if the solution appears homogenous, it's best to let it sit for a minute and see whether further layering occurs. If so, stir for a few more minutes. Check once more for separation before covering with plastic.

Problem: Alcohol stock becomes thick and gummy while cooking. Overevaporation of alcohol causes this problem.

Solution: Always weigh the pot before cooking. If the stock becomes frothy and gummy, weigh the pot again to determine just how much alcohol was lost. Replace the missing ounces with more alcohol.

Problem: White filmy residue floating on top of clearer soap solution. This film is composed of unsaponified fatty acids.

Solution: Either the soap needs more cooking, or the ingredients were mismeasured. In the case of mismeasurement, the mixture will need to be adjusted by the techniques given in Correcting Excess Fatty Acids on page 113.

A white film also develops when a wax such as lanolin is used, because of a high proportion of substances that do not saponify. In this case, no amount of cooking will change the soap's appearance. Shake these emollients into solution, or skim them off if you desire clear soap.

Problem: Cloudy soap. The causes of cloudy soap are many, as you will soon discover.

Solution: Prudent soapmakers will first dissolve an ounce of paste or alcohol-base soap in 2 ounces of hot water before diluting the entire 6-pound batch. If clouding appears after the sample solution has cooled (it often doesn't appear in a hot solution), you can still work with the paste or broth. You can't work with diluted soap. The presence of so much water effectively dampens any further chemical reactions between the oils and alkali.

Note: Please remember that initially undiluted soap (particularly when made with the paste method) will appear slightly cloudy because of insoluble fatty acids. These eventually precipitate out of solution. Don't interpret this kind of clouding as a sign of trouble. Learning to distinguish "good" clouding from "bad" is a matter of experience.

> **Alcohol boosts the rate of saponification.**

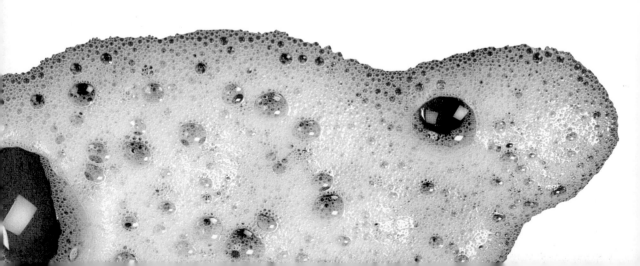

The Causes of Clouding

Clouding is a major concern for makers of liquid soap, and this problem can be caused by several factors. It will take a little trial and error for you to discover which cause is the culprit, but here is a guide to the most common causes.

▶ Oils or Additives.

Oils containing high percentages of palmitic or stearic acids form insoluble soaps, which in turn cause milkiness. Waxes such as lanolin and jojoba can cause clouding because of a high percentage of substances that do not saponify. Additives such as aloe vera juice and herbal infusions may be clear by themselves but can cloud when mixed with soap. Test everything possible in small samples, particularly additives, before compromising your entire batch of soap.

▶ Hard Water.

The minerals in hard water, particularly calcium, react with hydroxides to form insoluble mineral salts. Always use soft or distilled water.

▶ Insufficient Stirring of Paste.

Commercial potassium soaps are stirred constantly and cooked at very high temperatures. It's impossible to recreate these ideal conditions at home. A thoroughly mixed oil and lye solution, however, goes a long way toward ensuring a successful batch of soap. Stir until the emulsion turns into a thick glue, a sign that the oils and alkali are intimately mixed. Lighter, creamier emulsions may seem homogenous, but the oils and alkali won't be as intimately commingled. These lighter emulsions may not saponify properly. This problem might be corrected by cooking the paste for another hour or so. Otherwise, dissolve it in alcohol, and continue cooking until a test sample dissolved in water remains clear on cooling.

▶ Undercooking.

Generally, 3 hours for a paste and 2 hours for an alcohol soap broth is enough time to adequately neutralize all the fatty acids. But perhaps the water in the double boiler wasn't initially warm, or maybe the alcohol broth wasn't boiling throughout the 2 hours. Free fatty acids will be present in undercooked soap.

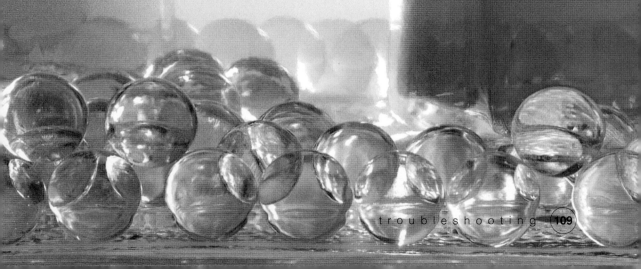

▶ Mismeasurement of Ingredients.

Excess fatty acids occur in liquid soap for any number of reasons, including understirring, undercooking, insufficient hydroxide, or excess oils. Too much oil or too little hydroxide from mismeasurement are the most common causes. Always double-check your weights. For correcting clouding caused by excess oil or insufficient alkali, consult Correcting pH Problems on page 112.

▶ Overaddition of Neutralizers.

Citric or boric acid will throw soap out of solution when added in excess, and this soap is further broken down into hydroxides and free fatty acids, causing cloudiness. Don't attempt to create a pH 7 commercial-style soap using these buffers; commercial "soaps" aren't soap. A pH 7 solution is possible if citric acid is added to true potassium soap, but by the time the pH is that low, the soap is no longer cloudy — instead, it actually "breaks" back into layers composed of oil and lye solution.

A soap solution can't be buffered below pH 9.5 with boric acid. Boric acid combines chemically with hydroxide to form potassium tetraborate, a cleansing, mild alkali. But even though the pH won't budge from a 9.5 reading, cloudiness increases with further additions of boric acid.

▶ **With careful planning and attention, you can avoid most, if not all, soapmaking problems.**

The clouding caused by excess neutralizer is probably best corrected by both the addition of solvents (alcohol, sugar, or glycerin) and a week or two of sequestering.

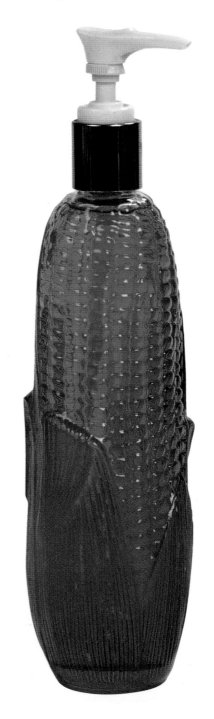

▶ Essential or Fragrance Oils.

Essential oils and fragrance oils aren't completely water soluble. It's important to add them to hot soap to optimize their dispersal. But some cloudiness will occur regardless, particularly with essential oils. A few days of sequestering usually clears the cloudiness caused by essential oils and fragrance oils. If this doesn't work, add a few ounces of solvent, such as glycerin, alcohol, or sugar solution, alone or in combination.

> Fragrance oils have been formulated with added solvents that aid in their dispersal. Most fragrance oils won't cloud soap to the extent that essential oils will.

▶ Excess Borax.

If your soap is too thin, you might be tempted to add a little extra borax for thickening. Try confining yourself to 2 to 3 percent (dry weight) borax per weight of diluted soap. Past that, you're bound to run into cloudiness because as the pH lowers, fatty acids are split from the soap. The best way to correct this problem is to thin the solution with some solvents, then sequester the soap for a week or two.

▶ Soap Solution Is Too Thick.

If the paste is made into a highly concentrated soap solution, cloudiness may occur; insoluble soaps are unable to precipitate out of solution because of the concentration of the liquid itself. This type of clouding is very minor, but if it bothers you, dilute the soap and sequester for a week or so until it is clear. Decant the clear liquid, then reheat the solution and evaporate it until the desired viscosity is achieved. Or add a few ounces of sequestrant.

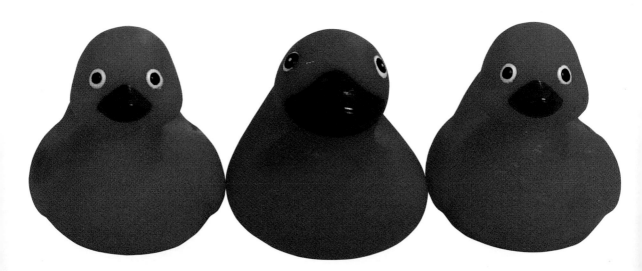

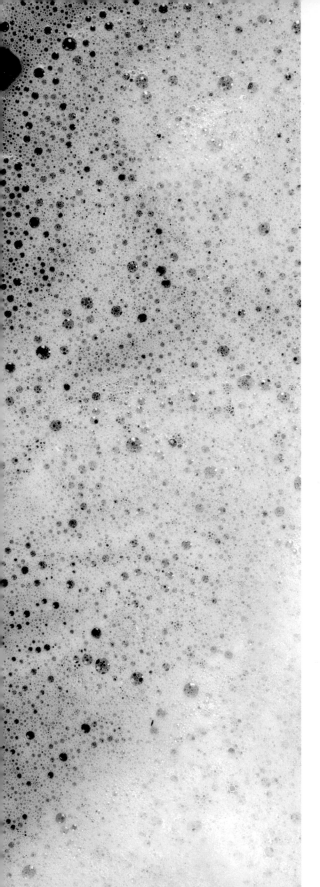

Correcting pH Problems

Phenolphthalein is practically indispensable for treating pH problems. A test solution of phenolphthalein turns clear in the presence of excess acid and changes to deep pink or red in the presence of excess alkali. It's that simple. Without it, you can only make educated guesses.

▶ **How to Test the pH.** For detailed instructions on using phenolphthalein to test the pH of your soap, see page 14.

What did the old-time soapmakers do before phenolphthalein? They used their tongues. If you don't have phenolphthalein, you might try their method. Using a very small amount of soap, lightly touch the cooled sample to the tip of the tongue. Neutral soap will have a mild bite, but only after several seconds. An immediate sharp sting indicates excess alkali. A very bland flavor with no bite at all indicates insufficient lye. This test is not very exact or scientific, but it may be better than nothing!

◀ Don't panic if you encounter a setback. Try one of the troubleshooting methods outlined here to correct a problem batch.

Correcting Excess Fatty Acids

Excess fatty acids can cause a soap to turn cloudy or form a film over the top. Fortunately, this problem can be fixed.

▶ How to Fix the Problem.

The first, and least painful, remedy for clouding caused by excess fatty acids is to cook the soap a little longer. The excess acids may just need more time in which to react with alkali. For pastes, another hour of cooking combined with some stirring should be sufficient. For alcohol-lye soaps, return the soap to the heat for another half hour.

After this additional cooking, withdraw an ounce of soap and dissolve it in 2 ounces of water. Allow the solution to cool. Is the soap sample still excessively cloudy? If so, stir the sample into an ounce of the phenolphthalein test solution. You know you have excess fatty acids in your soap when the faint pink of the test solution disappears. It's now time to add more hydroxide.

IN THE PINK

If a sample of cloudy soap solution turns the phenolphthalein test solution an even deeper shade of pink, this indicates that the soap contains excess alkali. In this case, more cooking is necessary, or additional oils might be needed.

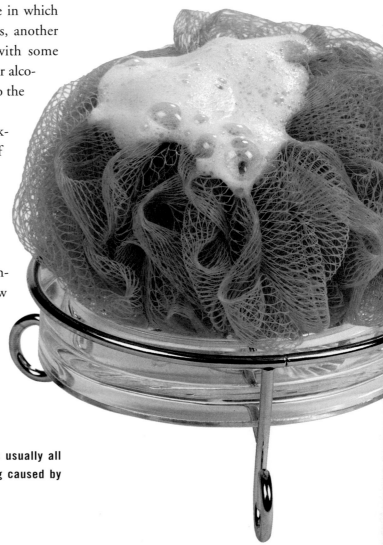

▶ A little extra cooking time is usually all that's needed to fix the clouding caused by excess fatty acids.

▶ **Add Hydroxide.** Create additional hydroxide solution by dissolving 2 ounces of dry hydroxide into 6 ounces of water (1:3 is the standard ratio for potassium solutions). The hydroxide must be blended into the soap, which is no problem if you're making the soap with the alcohol-lye method. But blending additional hydroxide into a tarlike paste is nearly impossible, so the paste must first be dissolved in 20 ounces of alcohol.

Now add 1 to 2 ounces of hydroxide solution, and cover the soap pot with plastic as instructed on page 34. Cook for another 20 to 30 minutes. Then withdraw another sample ounce of the soap, dissolve it in 2 ounces of water, and add to an ounce of phenolphthalein test solution. If the pink in the sample changes to clear, you know that more hydroxide is needed, so add another ounce or two of solution, and cook for another 20 minutes or so. Test again. Repeat this process until the phenolphthalein test solution remains faintly pink or a sample of soap dissolved in water exhibits only slight clouding when cooled.

If you don't have phenolphthalein, you'll need to rely on the appearance of the soap itself. Add an ounce or two of hydroxide solution according to the instructions above, cook for 20 to 30 minutes, then dissolve a 1-ounce test sample of soap in 2 ounces of water. Let cool. Does the solution still appear cloudy? If so, add another 1 to 2 ounces of hydroxide solution, and continue to cook. After 20 to 30 minutes, withdraw another 1-ounce sample, dissolve it in water, and cool. When the solution no longer clouds on cooling, your soap is ready to dilute and fragrance.

▼ **Give yourself a head start by becoming familiar with possible problems before you begin crafting.**

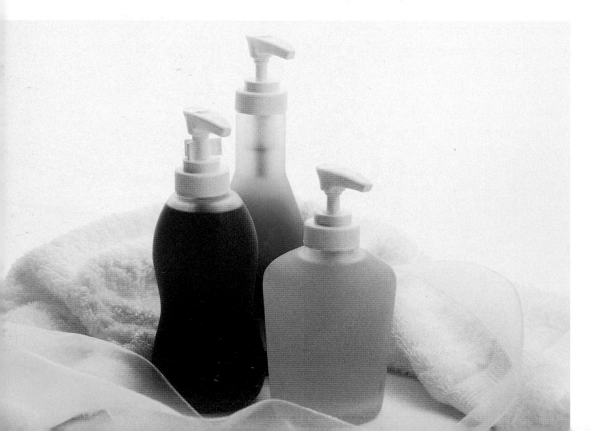

▶ Try Sequestering Agents.

Finally, if you don't want to recook your soap, consider adding sequestering agents, such as glycerin, alcohol, or sugar solution. In addition, let the soap sit for a week or two — much of the clouding may disappear. Remember, too, that cloudy soap is just as usable as clear soap, even though it may not be as aesthetically pleasing.

Correcting Excess Alkali

Soap contains excess alkali if 1 ounce of soap dissolved in 2 ounces of water registers a deeper pink when added to a phenolphthalein solution. The deeper the pink, the more alkaline the soap. Most likely, all samples will initially turn pink, because the formulations have been purposefully overalkalized. The addition of 8 to 12 drops of a 20 percent boric or citric acid solution should dissipate the pink. If a deep pink to red color remains, the soap is overalkaline.

If you don't have phenolphthalein, it may be difficult to diagnose overalkaline soap. Excess fatty acids manifest as a cloudiness in the soap, but excess alkali actually makes the soap clearer. (Keep in mind, however, that soap can be overalkaline as well as cloudy — an indication that it hasn't cooked long enough and that free fatty acids have yet to be neutralized.) Excess alkali can sometimes be spotted in the initial cooking phase of the paste, in such symptoms as a curdled emulsion or a paste that continues to puff up even after repeated stirrings. But not always.

So without phenolphthalein, you can always try the taste test mentioned on page 112. Excess hydroxide in the soap will register as an immediate sting on the tip of the tongue.

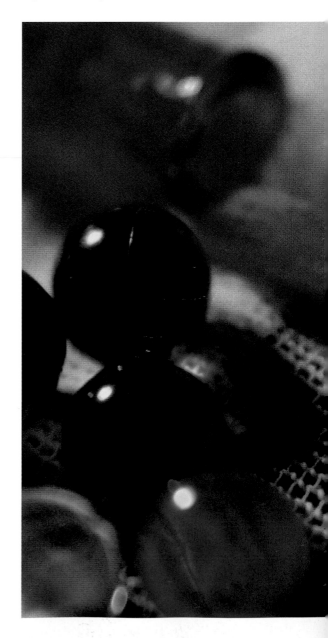

▶ **Use bath beads, colorful bottles and sponges, and tub toys to enhance your soap display.**

How to Remedy

The first course of action is to treat the overalkalinity as a problem stemming from undercooking. Return the paste to the heat for another hour; alcohol-based soap just needs another 30 or 40 minutes. After that, test a sample (1 ounce of soap dissolved in 2 ounces of water) in 1 ounce of phenolphthalein solution. Add 8 to 12 drops of citric or boric acid solution. If a deep pink color develops, it's time to add more oil.

Dissolve the paste in 20 ounces of alcohol; if you cooked the soap using the alcohol-lye method, you're all ready to add the oil. Add 1 to 2 ounces of castor oil to the solution, then cover with plastic according to the instructions outlined in The Alcohol/Lye Method on page 36. Return to the double boiler, and cook another 20 to 30 minutes. Test a sample (1 ounce of soap dissolved in 2 ounces of water) in 1 ounce of phenolphthalein solution. Add 8 to 12 drops of a 20 percent citric or boric acid solution. If a deep pink to red color again appears, additional castor oil will be needed. Add another ounce or two to the soap solution, cover, and continue cooking 20 to 30 more minutes. *Note:* More alcohol, too, may be necessary on account of the evaporation caused by extended cooking times.

Continue with this process until the phenolphthalein test solution remains a faint pink when soap solution is added.

> **Castor oil is the best oil for adjusting pH because it saponifies much more rapidly than other oils and helps impart clarity to the soap.**

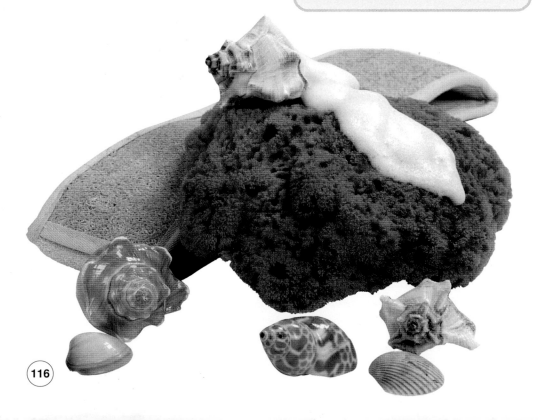

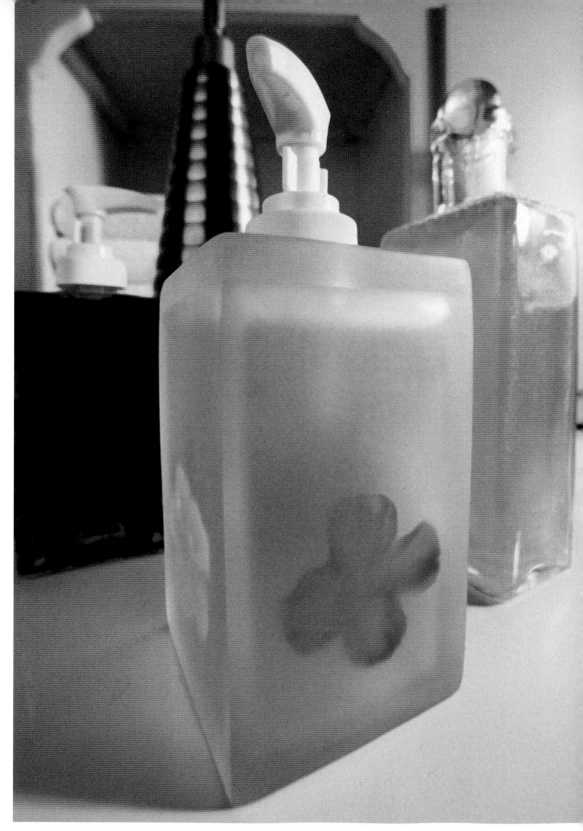

▶ After a little trial and error, you'll no doubt be creating flawless handmade soaps, shampoos, gels, and bubble baths.

Bibliography

Brannt, William. *The Soapmaker's Handbook*. Philadelphia: Henry Carey Baird Company, 1912.

Cavitch, Susan Miller. *The Soapmaker's Companion*. Pownal, VT: Storey Books, 1997.

"Fatty Acids and Liquid Soaps," *Emery Technical Bulletin*. Cincinnati, OH: Emery Industries, 1964.

Lamborn, Leebert. *Modern Soaps, Candles and Glycerin*. New York: Van Nostrand Company, 1906.

Milwidsky, B. "Soap and Detergent Technology," *Household and Personal Products Industries*. Ramsey, NJ: Rodman Publications, 1980.

Stanislaus, I. V. *American Soapmaker's Guide*. New York: Henry Carey Baird Company, 1928.

Thomssen, E. G., and Kemp, C. R. *Modern Soap Making*. New York: MacNair-Dorland Company, 1937.

Winter, Ruth. *A Consumer's Dictionary of Cosmetic Ingredients*. New York: Crown Publishers, Inc., 1984.

Glossary

Additive. A substance blended into finished soap to improve or fortify the soap. Sequestering agents, foam boosters, preservatives, and thickeners are all additives.

Alkali. Any base of hydroxide soluble in water and able to neutralize acids. In soapmaking, sodium or potassium hydroxide neutralizes fatty acids.

Borax, or sodium borate. A mild alkali used as a water softener, preservative, emulsifier, foam booster and stabilizer, pH buffer, and "viscosity modifier." One of the best all-around additives for liquid soap.

Cloud point. The point at which insoluble substances in a soap solution coalesce and cloud the solution. Solvents such as alcohol, glycerin, and sugar lower the cloud point, making it more difficult for these precipitates to coalesce. Chilling a soap solution will raise its cloud point, potentially causing clouding not present at room temperature.

Cold process. A soapmaking technique that relies almost exclusively on the heat generated by the chemical reaction of fatty acids and alkali to produce soap. No external heat is applied once the ingredients have been mixed.

Distilled water. Water that has been boiled, then condensed, to remove any minerals or other impurities.

Essential oil. A volatile oil steamed or pressed from the fruits, flowers, stems, or roots of plants. Used especially for perfumes, soaps, and flavoring.

Ethanol, or ethyl alcohol. Clear, colorless, and very flammable alcohol produced from the fermentation of carbohydrates. The primary alcohol used in the production of transparent soap.

Fatty acid. Any of the organic acids that, along with glycerides, are the main constituents of animal and vegetable fats and that react chemically with the alkalis to form soap. There are many kinds of fatty acids, and each has distinct properties that affect the characteristics of the soap produced from it.

Fragrance oil. A laboratory-produced synthetic version of a true essential oil or a natural fragrance, such as peach. Fragrance oils are often a combination of both synthetic and true essential oils.

Glycerin. A thick, sweet-tasting, clear fluid that's actually an alcohol. A by-product of soap manufacture, it can also be produced synthetically from propylene, a petroleum by-product. Used as an emollient, a humectant, and a primary solvent in the manufacture of transparent soaps.

Hard fat. Any animal or vegetable fat that is solid at room temperature; largely composed of the fatty acids stearin and palmitin. Palm oil and tallow are the two most common hard fats used for soapmaking.

Hot process. A soapmaking process whereby fats, oils, and a caustic solution are cooked at high temperatures over prolonged periods of time. The hot process is essential for all soaps in which clarity is desired, because high temperatures are needed to completely neutralize the excess fatty acids that cause cloudiness.

Humectant. A substance used to preserve moisture content.

Hydrogenation. The process of adding hydrogen gas to liquid oils. This process converts unsaturated fatty acids to their saturated analogs; oleic acid, for example, is converted to stearic acid. Hydrogenated oils can cause clouding in liquid soap.

Hydrolysis. From the Greek *hydro,* meaning "water," and *lysis,* "loosening." Hydrolysis is a form of decomposition through the chemical action of water. When fats or oils are mixed with a lye solution, hydrolysis causes fatty acids to separate from the glycerol.

Isopropyl alcohol. A petroleum-derived alcohol sometimes used as a substitute for ethanol. Isopropyl alcohol is an effective solvent and sequestering agent.

Lye. A very general term used to describe a strong alkaline solution. More specifically, lye solutions are composed of potassium hydroxide for liquid soap, or sodium hydroxide for bar soap.

pH. An abbreviation for the "potential of hydrogen," indicating acidity or alkalinity. A pH of 7, or the value of pure water, is regarded as neutral. Acids have a pH below 7; alkalis, above 7. "Neutral" soap, however, has a pH of approximately 9.5.

Phenolphthalein. A chemical compound used as an acid-base indicator.

Potassium carbonate. Also called pearl ash, this is a salt of potassium. When added to a potassium soap base, the molecules of pearl ash insert themselves between the molecules of potassium hydroxide, weakening the molecular pull between the hydroxide molecules. The result is softer, more stirrable soap paste.

Potassium hydroxide. A strong alkali also known as caustic potash. When combined with a fatty acid, it produces liquid soap.

Rosin. The pale yellow residue remaining after the volatile oils are distilled from the oleoresin of pine trees. Rosin is composed largely of abietic acid, which reacts with an alkali in much the same manner as fatty acids. Rosin adds transparency and emollience to a liquid soap, and acts as a preservative as well.

Saponification. The chemical reaction that converts a fatty acid and an alkali into soap and glycerin.

Sequester. This refers to the "resting phase" for the soap that lasts a week or two after dilution. During this time, any insoluble soaps can coalesce and precipitate out of solution. Sequestering improves the clarity of soap.

Sequestering agent. A soap additive that helps clarify the solution by lowering the cloud point. Alcohol, glycerin, and sugar solutions are all effective sequestering agents.

Soap. Along with glycerin, soap is the by-product of a chemical reaction involving fatty acids and caustic soda or potash. Soap is actually a salt.

Sodium hydroxide. Also known as caustic soda, it is one of two primary alkalis used in the production of soap. Combined with a fatty acid, it produces a hard soap.

Soft oil. Liquid at room temperature and characterized by a high percentage of oleic and linoleic unsaturated fatty acids. These fatty acids won't mar the clarity of the liquid. Castor oil is the soft oil of choice for transparent soapmaking because of its ability to act as a solvent; it is characterized by a high percentage of ricinoleic acid.

Solvent. A liquid capable of dissolving or dispersing another substance. Alcohol, glycerin, water, and sugar solutions are all solvents used to hold soap in a colloidal state for the purpose of rendering opaque soap transparent.

Sulfonated castor oil. Also called "turkey red oil," this oil is produced by the reaction of castor oil and sulfuric acid. Ideal for liquid soapmaking, it is a super-fatting agent that won't cause cloudiness, being completely water soluble.

Resources

Angel's Earth Natural Product Ingredients
1633 Scheffer Avenue
St. Paul, MN 55116-1427
(651) 698-3601
Fax: (651) 698-3636
E-mail: a-earth@pconline.com
Vegetable oils, sulfonated castor oil, jojoba, preservatives, essential and fragrance oils, dyes, lanolin, glycerin, citric acid, rosin, containers.

Aroma Creations, Inc.
24691 State Route 20
Sedro Woolley, WA 98284-8015
(360) 854-9000
Fax: (360) 856-4384
E-mail: aroma@gte.net
Fragrance oils, essential oils.

Aromystique, Inc.
P.O. Box 1482
Rockwall, TX 75087
(888) 722-1244
Fax: (972) 722-8082
Web site: www.aromystique.com
E-mail: dgutmann@aromystique.com
Vegetable oils, essential oils, containers.

Brambleberry
Bay Street Village
301 W. Holly, Suite M6
Bellingham, WA 98225
(360) 734-8278
Fax: (360) 738-5810
Web site: www.brambleberry.com
E-mail: bramblebery@prodigy.net
Preservatives, essential and fragrance oils, containers, glycerin, citric acid, soap molds, melt-and-pour supplies.

Camden-Grey Essential Oils
7178-A S.W. 47th Street
Miami, FL 33155
(877) 232-7662
Fax: (305) 740-8242
Web site: www.camdengrey.com
E-mail: info@camdengrey.com
Essential oils, vegetable oils, glycerin, citric acid, preservatives, containers.

Cat's Paw Enterprises
2333 Cape George Road
Port Townsend, WA 98368
(360) 385-3407
Contact person: Diana Johnson
Diana makes and sells goat milk soaps and water-based soaps. Her products cater to people with sensitive skin types and those with allergies.

Chem Lab Supplies
1060-C Ortega Way
Placentia, CA 92870
(714) 630-7902
Fax: (714) 630-3553
Web site: www.chemlab.com
E-mail: info@chemlab.com
Vegetable oils, sulfonated castor oil, lanolin, essential and fragrance oils, preservatives, dyes, glycerin, citric acid, sodium and potassium hydroxide, containers, phenolphthalein, rosin.

Country Scentuals
412 South Denny
Howe, TX 75459
(903) 532-2012
Web site: www.countryscentuals.com
E-mail: Reneerenee@aol.com
Contact person: Renee Thompson
Country Scentuals is an all-natural soap and toiletries company dedicated to creating the most luxurious bath products without the use of harsh chemicals.

Cranberry Lane Natural Beauty Products
65-2710 Barnet Highway
Coquitlam, B.C., Canada V3B1B8
(604) 944-1488
Fax: (604) 944-1439
Web site: www.cranberrylane.com
E-mail: staff@cranberrylane.com
Vegetable oils, rosin, sulfonated castor oil, essential oils, dyes, preservatives, glycerin, citric acid, phenolphthalein, containers, soap molds.

Delaware City Soap Company
P.O. Box 4112
Delaware City, DE 19706
(302) 832-7055
Web site: www.delcitysoap.com
E-mail: info@delcitysoap.com
Contact person: Rebecca Keilor
Located in a beautiful and historic riverfront town, this company specializes in authentic recreations of classic nineteenth-century soaps using fine vegetable ingredients and essential oils.

Designs By AnnaLiese
1430 N.W. 11th Street
Corvallis, OR 97330
Phone/fax: (541) 753-7881
E-mail: DesignsByA@aol.com
Contact person: AnnaLiese M. Moran
Custom soap design, soapmaking classes, and consulting.

The Essential Oil Company
1719 S.E. Umatilla Street
Portland, OR 97202
(800) 729-5912
Fax: (503) 872-8767
Web site: http://essentialoil.com
Vegetable oils, aromatherapy grade essential oils, fragrance oils, soapmaking supplies.

Flower Moon Soaps
8192 Bakers Lane
Chestertown, MD 21620
(410) 778-2385
Contact persons: Lisa and Matt Redman
Flower Moon Soaps makes soaps of unusual color and textures, using high-quality oils and a unique blending of fragrances for scents.

Frontier Natural Products Co-op
3021 78th Street
Norway, IA 52318
(800) 669-3275
Fax: (800) 717-4372
Web site: www.frontiercoop.com
E-mail: info@frontiercoop.com
Vegetable oils, essential and fragrance oils, lanolin, glycerin, dyes, preservatives, containers.

Georgie's Ceramic & Clay Co.
756 N.E. Lombard Street
Portland, OR 97211
(503) 283-1353
Web site: www.georgies.com
E-mail: alan@georgies.com
Contact person: John Alland
Fragrance oils, glycerin, dyes, containers, soap molds, melt-and-mold supplies. Check their Web site for information on their Eugene store.

Gingham 'n' Spice, Ltd./My Sweet Victoria
P.O. Box 88sm
Gardenville, PA 18926
(215) 348-3595
Fax: (215) 348-8021
Web site: www.fragrancesupplies.com
E-mail: mysweetvictoria@hotmail.com
Contact person: Nancy Booth
Bottles, bulk oils, glycerin, cocoa butter, beeswax pearls, kaolin clay, colorants, mica.

Herbal Accents
P.O. Box 937
Alpine, CA 91903-0937
(888) 440-4380
Fax: (760) 632-7279
Web site: www.herbalaccents.com
E-mail: herbal@herbalaccents.com
Vegetable oils, essential and fragrance oils, potassium hydroxide, glycerin, herbal extracts, butter, citric acid, preservatives, dyes, containers, melt-and-pour supplies.

Homesong Handcrafted Soaps
5220 Zimmer Road
Williamston, MI 48895
(517) 655-4037
Web site: www.MIcrafts.com
E-mail: Trish4000@ aol.com
Contact person: Trisha Walton

Indiana Botanic Gardens
3401 W. 37th Avenue
Hobart, IN 46342
(888) 315-3077 (wholesale)
(800) 644-8327
Fax: (219) 947-4148
Web site: www.botanichealth.com
E-mail: info@botanichealth.com
Vegetable oils, fragrance and essential oils.

Indian River Creations
1478 Highland Avenue
Melbourne, FL 32935
(800) 686-7362
Fax: (321) 255-7245
Web site: www.indianriversoap.com
E-mail: sales@indianriversoap.com
Contact person: Debby Graybeal
Every uniquely scented soap from Indian River Creations has a purpose, including antibacterial, disinfecting, relaxing, or energizing.

Iowa Natural Soapworks
911 W. 16th Street
Davenport, IA 52804
Voice/fax/orders: (800) 265-5252
Web site: www.IowaNaturalSoapworks.com
E-mail: jasidney@netexpress.net
Contact person: Jill Sidney
Iowa Natural Soapworks soap is a high-quality, handcrafted, natural soap.

Janca's Jojoba Oil & Seed Co.
456 E. Juanita #7
Mesa, AZ 85204
(480) 497-9494
Fax: (480) 497-1312
E-mail: Jancas3@aol.com
Vegetable oils, essential and fragrance oils, potassium hydroxide, sulfonated castor oil, glycerin, citric acid, preservatives, containers.

Liberty Natural Products
8120 S.E. Stark Street
Portland, OR 97215
(800) 298-8427
Fax: (503) 256-1182
Web site: www.libertynatural.com
E-mail: sales@libertynatural.com
Vegetable oils, essential oils, sulfonated castor oil, preservatives, glycerin, citric acid, dyes, containers, soap molds, melt-and-pour supplies.

LorAnn Oils Inc.
4518 Aurelius Road
Lansing, MI 48909
Mailing address:
P.O. Box 22009
Lansing, MI 48909
(888) 456-7266
Fax: (517) 882-0507
Web site: www.lorannoils.com
Vegetable oils, sulfonated castor oil, essential and fragrance oils, rosin, glycerin, citric acid.

Majestic Mountain Sage
881 West 700 North Suite 107
Logan, UT 84321
(435) 755-0863
Fax: (435) 755-2108
Web site: www.the-sage.com
E-mail: info@the-sage.com
Vegetable oils, fragrance and essential oils, phenolph-thalein, glycerin, citric acid, dyes, containers.

Milky Way Molds
PMB #473
4326 S.E. Woodstock
Portland, OR 97206
(800) 588-7930
(503) 774-4157
Fax: (503) 777-6584
Web site: www.milkywaysoapmolds.com
E-mail: sales@milkywaysoapmolds.com
Soap molds, soap stamps.

Natural Impulse Handmade Soap and Sundries
P.O. Box 94441
Birmingham, AL 35220-4441
(877) IMPULSE
Web site: www.naturalimpulse.com
E-mail: sales@naturalimpulse.com
Contact person: Karen White
Natural Impulse sells luxurious handmade soaps and toiletries, and offers a free weekly Internet column on the soapmaking business. For more information, see the Web site.

North Country Mercantile
Box 5368
West Lebanon, NH 03784
(603) 795-2843
Web site: www.northcountrymercantile.com
E-mail: northcountry@esosoft.com
Vegetable oils, essential and fragrance oils, containers, soap molds.

Nurnberg Scientific
6310 S.W. Virginia
Portland, OR 97201
(503) 246-8297
Fax: (503) 246-0360
Web site: www.nurnberg.com
E-mail: sales@nurnberg.com
Vegetable oils, essential and fragrance oils, glycerin, potassium hydroxide, rosin, preservatives, phenolphthalein.

Penta Manufacturing Co., Inc.
50 Okner Parkway
Livingston, NJ 07039-1604
(973) 740-2300
Fax: (973) 740-1839
Web site: www.pentamfg.com
E-mail: sales@pentamfg.com
Vegetable oils, essential oils, glycerin, potassium and sodium hydroxide, glycerin, citric acid, preservatives.

Pharmco Products, Inc.
58 Vale Road
Brookfield, CT 06804-3967
(800) 243-5360
Fax: (203) 740-3481
Web site: www.pharmco-prod.com
E-mail: pharmco@pharmco-prod.com
5-gallon containers of SDA-3A (denatured alcohol), 1 per year without permit.

Pisces Rising Aromatherapy Arts and Crafts
1631 N. Colorado
Indianapolis, IN 46218
(317) 375-1718
Web site: http://pages.prodigy.net/ewinslow/
   pisces.htm
E-mail: ewinslow@prodigy.net
Contact person: Ethel Winslow
Pisces Rising Aromatherapy Arts and Crafts was established in 1993 to provide all-natural personal care products and educate the public about aromatherapy.

Poya Naturals Inc.
21–B Regan Road
Brampton, Ontario, Canada L7A 1C5
(877) 255-7692
Fax: (905) 846-1784
Web site: www.poyanaturals.com
E-mail: deccan@interlog.com
Essential oils.

Pretty Baby Herbal Soap Company
P.O. Box 555
China Grove, NC 28023
Web site: www.prettybabysoap.com
(800) 673-8167
Soapmaking kits, supplies.

Rainbow Meadow Inc.
8433 South Avenue, Suite 2
Poland, OH 44512
(800) 207-4047
Fax: (517) 764-0940
Web site: www.rainbowmeadow.com
Vegetable oils, essential oils, glycerin, citric acid, preservatives, dyes, containers, phenolphthalein, soap molds, melt-and-pour supplies.

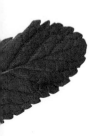
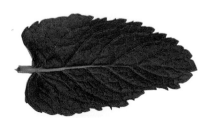

Robert and Katherine McDaniel
3550 Val Verde Avenue
Long Beach, CA 90808
(562) 761-5311
E-mail: bobnkate@earthlink.net
Contact person: Bob McDaniel
Robert and Katherine McDaniel features Dr. Bob's Herbal Soaps, made from skin-friendly aromatherapy-type oils, bath salts, and powders.

Scentsables
23813 N.E. Canyon Loop
Battle Ground, WA 98604
(360) 687-3502
Web site: www.angelfire.com/biz/
    NaturalSoaps/index.html
E-mail: naturalsoaps@angelfire.com
Contact person: Maggie Anderson
Scentsables creates herbal and vegetable-based soaps in small batches using the cold-process method. Many contain fragrant ground herbs, herbal extracts, and essential oils.

Serenity Soaps and Herb Gardens
630 Dodge Road
Camano Island, WA 98282
Phone/fax: (360) 387-0727
E-mail: serenityherbs@yahoo.com
Contact person: Sharon Dodge

Shay & Co., Inc.
7941 Southeast Steele Street, Suite 2
Portland, OR 97206
(503) 775-3420
Fax: (503) 775-3486
Web site: www.shayandcompany.com
E-mail: wshay@teleport.com
Vegetable oils, preservatives, melt-and-pour supplies, soapmaking supplies.

Simple Pleasures
P.O. Box 194
Old Saybrook, CT 06475
Phone/fax: (860) 395-0085
Web site: http://members.aol.com/pigmntlady/
E-mail: PigmntLady@aol.com
Pigments, dyes.

Snowdrift Farm Natural Products
3759 North Romero Road, Suite 141
Tucson, AZ 85705
(888) 999-6950
Web site: www.snowdriftfarm.com
E-mail: info@snowdriftfarm.com
Contact names: Bill and Trina Wallace
Snowdrift Farm provides handmade soaps from all-natural products, as well as supplying essential oils and raw materials to soap and toiletry makers. They carry vegetable oils, essential oils, potassium hydroxide, citric acid, dyes, and containers.

SoapBerry Lane
P.O. Box 65551
Virginia Beach, VA 23467
Phone/fax: (757) 490-8852
Web site: www.soapberrylane.com
E-mail: soapberyln@aol.com
Dyes, glycerin, fragrance oils, soap molds, melt-and-pour supplies, liquid silk, pumice, and more.

The Soap Box
424 Third Street West
Cochrane, Alberta, Canada T4C 1Z6
(403) 932-4530
Web site: www.thesoapbox.org
E-mail: customde@cadvision.com
Contact person: Donna Ramsey
The Soap Box sells soapmaking kits, fizzy-o-therapy (bath bombs), lotions, lip balms, cold-process soaps, shower gels, and shampoos. They have training programs to teach people how to use the soapmaking kits.

Soap Crafters Company
2944 S.W. Temple
Salt Lake City, UT 84115
(801) 484-5121
Fax: (801) 487-1958
Web site: www.soapcrafters.com
E-mail: pam@soapcrafters.com
Vegetable oils, fragrance oils, soap molds, melt-and-pour supplies.

Soaper's Choice
A division of:
Columbus Foods
730 North Albany Avenue
Chicago, IL 60612
(800) 322-6457
Fax: (773) 265-6985
Web site: www.soaperschoice.com
Contact person: Mike Lawson
Base oils and vegetable glycerin soap bases for all your soapmaking needs.

The Soap Saloon
5710 Auburn Boulevard #6
Sacramento, CA 95841
(916) 334-4894
Fax: (916) 334-4897
Web site: www.soapsaloon.com
Vegetable oils, essential and fragrance oils, glycerin, citric acid, preservatives, dyes, soap molds.

Soapscope Inc.
828 College Street
Toronto, Ontario, Canada M6G 1C8
(888) 340-5877
Fax: (416) 588-8734
Web site: www.soapscope.com
E-mail: soap@soapscope.com
Palm oil, essential and fragrance oils, citric acid, soap molds, melt-and-pour supplies.

Stevenson-Cooper, Inc.
1039 W. Venango Street
P.O. Box 46345
Philadelphia, PA 19160
(888) 420-1663
E-mail: waxcooper@aol.com
Fax: (215) 223-3597
Vegetable oils, tallow, rosin.

Sugar Plum Sundries
1715 East Main Street
Chattanooga, TN 37404
Phone/fax: (423) 624-4511
Web site: www.sugarplum.net
E-mail: info@sugarplum.net
Vegetable oils, essential oils, potassium hydroxide, citric acid, preservatives.

Summers Past Farms Ye Olde Soap Shoppe
15602 Olde Highway 80
Flinn Springs, CA 92021
(619) 390-3525
Fax: (619) 390-7148
Web site: www.soapmaking.com
E-mail: farmsup@aol.com
Vegetable oils, fragrance and essential oils, potassium hydroxide, glycerin, citric acid, preservatives, dyes, soap molds, containers.

SunCoast Soaps & Supplies
12415 Haley Street
Sun Valley, CA 91352
(818) 252-1452
Fax: (818) 252-1034
E-mail: info@suncoastsoaps.com
Soapamking supplies, fragrance oils, shrink wrap machines.

Sunfeather Natural Soap Co.
1551 State Highway 72
Potsdam, NY 13676
(315) 265-3648
Fax: (315) 265-2902
Web site: www.sunsoap.com
E-mail: sunsoap@slic.com
Vegetable oils, essential oils, glycerin, preservatives, dyes, soap molds.

Sweet Cakes Soapmaking Supplies
18 North Road
Kinnelon, NJ 07405
(973) 838-5200
Fax: (973) 838-9925
Web site: www.sweetcakes.com
E-mail: sweetcakes@nac.net
Fragrance oils, glycerin soap base, soap molds.

TKB Trading
356 24th Street
Oakland, CA 94612
(510) 451-9011
Fax: (510) 839-9967
Web site: www.tkbtrading.com
E-mail: tkbtrading@aol.com
Vegetable oils, essential and fragrance oils, glycerin, rosin, sulfonated castor oil, preservatives, dyes, citric acid, phenolphthalein, containers, soap molds, melt-and-pour supplies.

Tom Thumb Workshops
59 Market Street
Onancock, VA 23417
(800) 526-6502
Fax: (757) 787-3136
Web site: www.tomthumbworkshops.com
E-mail: ttw@esva.net
Vegetable oils, essential and fragrance oils, containers, glycerin soap base, colorants, reference materials.

Uncommon Scents
P.O. Box 1941
Eugene, OR 97440
(514) 345-0952
Fax: (888) 343-8196
Web site: www.uncommonscents.com
E-mail: sales@uncommonscents.com
Vegetable oils, essential and fragrance oils, preservatives, containers.

Wholesale Supplies Plus, Inc.
13390 York Road Unit G
North Royalton, OH 44133
(800) 359-0944
Fax: (440) 237-0639
Web site: www.wholesalesuppliesplus.com
E-mail: SoapPlus@aol.com
Essential and fragrance oils, glycerin, dyes, containers, soap molds, melt-and-pour supplies.

Zenith Supplies
6300 Roosevelt Way N.E.
Seattle, WA 98115
(206) 525-7997
Fax: (206) 525-3703
Web site: www.zenithsupplies.com
Vegetable oils, essential and fragrance oils, glycerin, citric acid, dyes, containers, soap molds, melt-and-pour supplies.

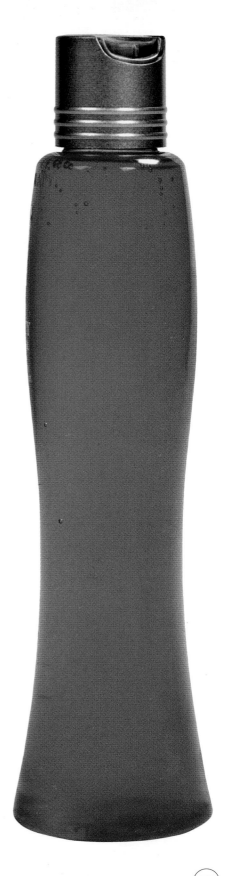

Index

CONVERTING RECIPE MEASUREMENTS TO METRIC

Use the following chart for converting U.S. measurements to metric. Since the conversions are not exact, it's important to convert the measurements for all of the ingredients to maintain the same proportions as the original recipe.

To convert to	When the measurement given is	Multiply it by
milliliters	teaspoons	4.93
milliliters	tablespoons	14.79
milliliters	fluid ounces	29.57
milliliters	cups	236.59
liters	cups	0.236
milliliters	pints	473.18
liters	pints	0.473
milliliters	quarts	946.36
liters	quarts	0.946
liters	gallons	3.785
grams	ounces	28.35
kilograms	pounds	0.454
centimeters	inches	2.54
degrees Celsius	degrees Fahrenheit	$\frac{5}{9}\,(°-32)$

Other Storey Books You Will Enjoy

Making Transparent Soap, by Catherine Failor. A colorful, comprehensive, step-by-step guide to creating homemade transparent soaps. Includes thorough instructions for making, coloring, scenting, and molding these popular bar soaps. 144 pages. Paperback. ISBN 1-58017-244-X.

The Soapmaker's Companion, by Susan Miller Cavitch. The most authoritative guide ever written on making natural, vegetable-based soaps. In addition to basic soapmaking instructions, readers will learn how to use specialty techniques and make transparent, liquid, and imprinted soaps. Includes information on chemistry, ingredients, additives, colorants, and scents. 288 pages. Paperback. ISBN 0-88266-965-6.

The Handmade Soap Book, by Melinda Coss. Using step-by-step instructions and full-color photographs, you can craft a wide variety of bath products from one basic recipe. Create your own unique soaps by experimenting with natural colorings, textures, and scents. 80 pages. Hardcover. ISBN 1-58017-084-6.

Milk-Based Soaps, by Casey Makela. Makela shares her simple technique for making moisturizing milk-based soaps. Covers making classic beauty soaps and specialty soaps, as well as how to turn this hobby into a moneymaker. 112 pages. Paperback. ISBN 0-88266-984-2.

The Natural Soap Book, by Susan Miller Cavitch. An inspiring exploration of the goodness of soap without chemical additives and synthetic ingredients. Step-by-step instructions for creating basic vegetable-based soaps plus suggestions for scenting, coloring, cutting, and wrapping are included. 192 pages. Paperback. ISBN 0-88266-888-9.

The Essential Oils Book, by Colleen K. Dodt. A rich resource on the many applications of aromatherapy and its uses in everyday life, including aromas for the home, scents for business environments, and essences for the elderly. 160 pages. Paperback. ISBN 0-88266-913-3.

The Herbal Body Book, by Stephanie Tourles. Learn how to transform common herbs, fruits, and grains into safe, economical, and natural personal-care items. Contains more than 100 recipes for facial scrubs, hair rinses, shampoos, soaps, cleansing lotions, moisturizers, lip balms, toothpaste, powders, and more! 128 pages. Paperback. ISBN 0-88266-880-3.

The Herbal Home Spa, by Greta Breedlove. These easy-to-make recipes include facial steams, scrubs, masks, and lip balms; massage oils, baths, rubs, and wraps; hand, nail, and foot treatments; and shampoos, dyes, and conditioners. 208 pages. Paperback. ISBN 0-88266-005-6.

These books and other Storey books are available at your bookstore, farm store, or garden center, or directly from Storey Books, 210 MASS MoCA Way, North Adams, MA 01247, or by calling 1-800-441-5700. Or visit our Web site at www.storey.com.

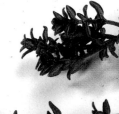